Biosafety
Reference Manual

Second Edition

Prepared by the
American Industrial Hygiene Association
Biosafety Committee

Edited by Patricia A. Heinsohn, Robert R. Jacobs,
and Beth A. Concoby

ISBN 0-932627-65-X

American Industrial Hygiene Association
2700 Prosperity Avenue, Suite 250
Fairfax, VA 22031
Stock No. 204-RC-95

Contributors

Beth A. Concoby, CIH,
Genencor International, S. San Francisco, CA

Daniel A. Ghidoni, PE, CIH, CSP
The Baker Company, Sanford, ME

Marc A. Gomez, CIH, CSP,
N. Broward Hospital District, Fort Lauderdale, FL

Patricia A. Heinsohn, Ph.D., CIH,
Clayton Environmental Consultants, Pleasanton, CA

Robert R. Jacobs, Ph.D.,
School of Public Health, University of Alabama-Birmingham, Birmingham, AL

Joseph K. Kwan, D. Env., CIH,
Hong Kong University of Science and Technology, Kowloon, Hong Kong

Daniel F. Liberman, Ph.D.,
Boston University Medical Center, Boston, MA

Vernon E. Rose, Dr PH, CIH,
School of Public Health, University of Alabama-Birmingham, Birmingham, AL

James S. Spahr, MPH, RS,
Phoenix Indian Medical Center, Phoenix, AZ

Contents

Figures

Tables

1. Introduction

This guide was prepared by the American Industrial Hygiene Association Biosafety Committee. As a technical committee duly constituted by the AIHA Board of Directors, we are providing information we hope will help in addressing questions about biohazards in the workplace.

The intent of this manual is not to cover all occupational settings or all biohazardous agents. A few occupational settings — namely laboratory, health care, and biotechnology — are discussed. Bloodborne pathogens, tuberculosis, biogenic toxins, and allergens are discussed in depth. Our intent is to provide the reader with basic information on biohazards and the control of biohazard exposures that can be applied despite the occupational setting and biohazards involved.

For the purposes of this publication, a biohazardous agent is one of biological origin that has the capacity to produce deleterious effects on humans. Occupational biohazards include those organisms or substances of biological origin that occur in the working environment and cause — or have the potential to cause — deleterious effects on exposed workers or their families. Included in this definition are viable microorganisms and toxins and allergens derived from these organisms; arthropods, including species that might directly cause adverse effects (a bite or sting) or might produce substances that act as an allergen or toxin; and allergens and toxins derived from higher plants and animals.

The presence of an organism or biologically derived substance in the work environment does not necessarily represent a hazard. The hazard potential depends on a complex relationship between agent factors, host factors, and work environmental factors. Each of these factors must be considered when assessing the health risk potential from biological agents.

The definition of biosafety is also important. Biosafety is used in this manual to describe a complete program of administrative controls, medical surveillance, vaccination, and containment strategies for reducing the risk of disease in employees facing potential occupational exposure to infectious agents or other biologically derived molecules.

This publication is organized as follows: The first three chapters provide background information about the three types of responses generally associated with exposure to biohazardous agents: infections, intoxications, and allergic responses. Within these three chapters, more detailed information is provided in sections that focus on either specific biohazardous materials, environments, or sampling methodologies that are pertinent to that chapter. The objective of the detailed treatment is to provide the practicing industrial hygienist or occupational health and safety professional with sufficient information to allow them to anticipate some of the difficulties of biohazard remediation. It will help them tailor a biosafety program that addresses their specific needs.

In addition to chapters covering the specific types of responses to biohazardous agents, there are two chapters that generically address control strategies and methods for the decontamination, disinfection, sterilization, and handling of biohazardous waste.

Although the AIHA Biosafety Committee believes this manual provides a comprehensive overview of biosafety, the committee recommends that other resources be consulted in developing a biosafety program. Table I contains a list of published biosafety guidelines, and Appendix I is a bibliography of literature pertaining to issues in biosafety.

Table I. Other Published Biosafety Guidelines

Title	Issued by	Date Published
Laboratory Safety Monograph	U.S. Department of Health, Education and Welfare, National Institutes of Health	January 2, 1979
Laboratory Biosafety Manual	World Health Organization	1983
Recombinant DNA Laboratory Manual	Academic Press, San Diego	1984
Points to Consider in the Production and Testing of New Drugs and Biologicals Produced by Recombinant DNA Technology	U.S. Food and Drug Administration, Office of Biologics Research and Review, Center for Drugs and Biologics	April 10, 1985
"Coordinated Framework for Regulation of Biotechnology," Federal Register 51(123): 23301-23750 (1986)	Office of Science and Technology Policy	June 26, 1986
Recombinant DNA Safety Considerations	Organisation for Economic Co-operation and Development	July 16, 1986
EPA Guide for Infectious Waste Management	U.S. Environmental Protection Agency	1986
Laboratory Safety: Principles and Practices	American Society of Microbiology	1986
Manual of Industrial Microbiology	American Society of Microbiology	1986
Protection of Laboratory Workers from Infectious Disease Transmitted by Blood and Tissue (Proposed Guidelines)	National Committee for Clinical Laboratory Standards (NCCLS), Document #M-29-P	1987
Points to Consider in the Characterization of Cell Lines Used to Produce Biologicals	U.S. Food and Drug Administration, Office of Biologics Research and Review, Center for Drugs and Biologics	1987
Points to Consider in the Manufacture and Testing of Monoclonal Antibody Products for Human Use	U.S. Food and Drug Administration, Office of Biologics Research and Review, Center for Drugs and Biologics	1987
Biosafety in Microbiological and Biomedical Laboratories	U.S. Department of Health and Human Services	May, 1988
Protection of Laboratory Workers from Infectious Disease Transmitted by Blood and Tissue (Tentative Guidelines)	National Committee for Clinical Laboratory Standards	January, 1989
Biosafety in the Laboratory	National Academy of Science	1989/1990
Categorization of Pathogens According to Hazards and Categories of Containment	Advisory Committee on Dangerous Pathogens. London: HMSO	1990
Bloodborne Pathogens Standard (29 CFR 1910.1030)	U.S. Department of Labor, Occupational Safety and Health Administration	1992
Guidelines for Research Involving Recombinant DNA Molecules (NIH Guidelines)	U.S. Department of Health and Human Services, National Institutes of Health	June 1994
Protection of Laboratory Workers from Instrumental Biohazards	National Committee for Clinical Laboratory Standards, Document #117-P	N/A

N/A = not available

2. Viable Microorganisms

A. Overview

1. Basic Microbiology

Of the thousands of microbes inhabiting our earth, only a small fraction is pathogenic to man. Included in this group of medically important microorganisms are viruses, bacteria, chlamydiae, rickettsiae, mycoplasmas, and fungi. However, in addition to pathogenic species, free-living or saprophytic microorganisms may represent a health risk under conditions of intense exposure or to susceptible (e.g., immunocompromised) individuals.

Industrial hygienists involved in biohazard analysis need to understand the dynamics of microorganisms in various occupational settings before they can effectively design control measures to prevent occupational infections. Each organism requires a set of parameters for its growth, metabolism, development, and reproduction. The external environment must provide favorable conditions for the maintenance of these internal vital processes before the organism can successfully compete with other microbes and be able to survive and grow in the particular environment.

Environmental factors that might affect the survival of microbes include moisture content, temperature, acidity/alkalinity, osmotic pressure, oxygen tension, nutrients, and lighting. Organism characteristics such as the presence of environmentally resistant capsules and virulence factors often determine the survivability of the organism and its ability to cause disease in the host. A thorough understanding of these issues may be acquired by consulting a current textbooks in microbiology.[1]

Viruses are submicroscopic, subcellular, filterable agents consisting of a central core of nucleic acid wrapped in a protective coat of protein that may, in turn, be surrounded by a lipoprotein membrane. The nucleic acid of a virus is either DNA (deoxyribonucleic acid) or RNA (ribonucleic acid). Viruses do not have energy generating and biosynthesis mechanisms. Their replication requires the active participation of host cells. The size of viruses ranges between 0.02–0.3 μm. Electron microscopy has shown that viruses occur in different shapes, with some taking the shape of spheres, rods, bricks, bullets and tadpoles. Viruses are classified according to their size, morphology, symmetry, kind of nucleic acid, and ether stability (which is an indicator of the lipid content of the protective coat).

Bacteria appear in many different sizes and shapes. Their morphological features have been used for grouping purposes. Representative spheroidal or coccal shaped bacteria include the *Staphylococcus* and *Streptococcus* species. Cylindrical or rod shaped organisms include the *Escherichia* and *Salmonella* species. Curved rods are exemplified by the *Vibrio* genus (the causative agent for cholera) and the coiled thread-like organisms are exemplified by the *Treponema* genus (causative agent for syphilis). Filamentous bacteria are represented by the *Actinomycete* genus. The majority of bacteria measure between 0.5–1.0 μm × 2–5 μm.

Another way of classifying bacteria is by the use of staining reactions, which are based on the reaction between certain dyes and the bacterial cell wall components. One commonly used staining procedure is the Gram stain. This reaction depends on the fact that when certain bacteria are stained with an aniline dye (such as gentian violet) and are subsequently fixed with a potassium iodide solution, treatment with alcohol fails to decolorize the bacteria. Other bacteria, after going through the same procedure, are readily decolorized. Bacteria that are able to retain the color are called Gram-positive (GPB); those that are unable to retain the color are called Gram-negative (GNB).

The differences in the staining characteristics of GNB and GPB are in the chemical composition and structure of the cell wall. A variety of other staining procedures can be used to enhance the microscopic examination of bacteria. These procedures may yield information on size, shape, staining reaction, spore formation, motility, and capsule formation.

Microscopically, bacteria can be visualized as "colonies" on culture media. When bacteria are seeded sparsely over the surface of solid media, the individual organisms multiply and form isolated colonies, termed a colony forming unit (CFU). The appearance of the colonies are often characteristic of particular species. In addition to physical properties, bacteria can also be identified by biochemical and serological reactions.

Chlamydiae, such as the causative agent for trachoma (*Chlamydia trachoma*), measure 0.25–0.5 μm in diameter. They are obligate intracellular parasites that multiply by means of a unique developmental cycle. They produce characteristic cytoplasmic inclusions in susceptible host cells. They are susceptible to antimicrobials such as sulfonimides, chloramphenicol, and tetracycline. They possess group specific complement-fixing antigens. Individual members are identified by their virulence for different hosts, by the pathology produced and by the possession of specific antigens.

Rickettsiae are small pleomorphic coccobacilli that can only multiply within susceptible host cells. Most of them require an arthropod host for perpetuation in nature. Although rickettsiae and bacteria are very similar in morphology and metabolic characteristics, most rickettsiae possess cell membranes that are permeable to metabolites, such as nucleotides. This leakage of nucleotides into the environment may be the basis for their lability and failure to multiply outside of the susceptible host cells. *Coxiella burnetti*, the causative agent for Q fever, is an important exception. It survives well in the environment.

Mycoplasmas are the smallest cells capable of independent existence. Some are smaller than the larger viruses and can pass through filters with an average pore size of 0.15 μm. They differ from bacteria in the absence of a cell wall and in the presence of sterols in the cell membrane. Therefore, they are not susceptible to antibiotics that interfere with cell wall synthesis. *Mycoplasma pneumonia* is the causative agent for primary atypical pneumonia.

Fungi can exists either in the yeast or mold phase depending upon environmental conditions. Yeast are unicellular, oval cells 3–5 μm in diameter. Molds consists mainly of long branching filaments known as hyphae which are tubular structure 2–10 μm in diameter. Hyphae consist of several cells lying end to end, usually separated from one another by septa. A mass of intertwining hyphae is known as a "mycelium." Yeast cells reproduce by budding, but molds reproduce by apical growth of hyphae, by formation of spores, or by fragmentation of hyphae. Some species are even capable of sexual reproduction similar to those of higher plants. The spores are highly resistant to adverse environmental conditions and can germinate under favorable conditions to give rise to new colonies of hyphae.

"Mycoses" is the term used to describe fungal infections in man. They are classified as systemic, subcutaneous, and superficial mycoses. Fungi capable of causing systemic infection include *Coccidioides immitis* (San Joaquin Valley Fever), and *Histoplasma capsulatum* (found in pigeon droppings). *Sporotrichum schenckii* is the only important fungus causing subcutaneous mycosis. Genera capable of causing superficial infection include *Microsporum*, *Trichophyton*, and *Epidermophyton*.

Besides being capable of causing infections, some fungi have been demonstrated to cause allergenic responses such as hypersensitivity pneumonitis. Examples of these organisms include the saprophytes *Cladosporium*, *Aspergillus*, and *Alternaria*.

2. Routes of Exposure

In the occupational environment, significant routes of exposure to infectious agents include ingestion, inhalation, inoculation, skin and mucous membrane penetration, and animal and insect bites.

Ingestion of pathogenic microbes occurs frequently as results of poor personal hygiene and poor laboratory practice. Handling infectious materials without gloves and failure to wash contaminated hands before handling food are some common mistakes. Eating, drinking, smoking, and application of cosmetics or contact lenses in laboratories also can result in ingestion of infectious agents and exposure to the conjunctiva.

Inhalation exposure occurs when aerosol generating procedures are conducted in an open area without containment. Operations such as centrifugation, sonication, homogenization, and mixing generate aerosols. These operations must be conducted in controlled environments to prevent employee exposure.

Inoculation frequently occurs as accidental injections with contaminated needles or cuts with contaminated sharp instruments. Inadequate control of infected experimental animals and infected insect vectors may also result in the infection of the laboratory worker through accidental bites.

Although all of these routes account for a percentage of known infections, inhalation probably accounts for the majority of all occupational infections. Many laboratory operations produce aerosol.

Table II provides data from a series of air-sampling determinations showing the numbers of viable particles generated by standard laboratory operations.[2,3]

Table II. Concentration and Particle Size of Aerosols Created During Named Laboratory Techniques [A]

	Number of Viable Colonies [B]	Particle Size in Micrometers [C]
Mixing culture w/ pipet	6.0	3.5
Mechanical mixer for 15 seconds	0	0
Mixer overflow	9.4	4.8
Use of blender		
w/ top on during operation	119	1.9
w/ top removed after operation	1500	1.7
Use of sonicator	6	4.8
Lyophylized cultures		
Opened carefully	134	10.0
Dropped	4838	10.0

[A] Source: **Kenny, M.T., and F.L. Sabel:** Particle Size Distribution of *Serratia marcescens* Aerosols Created During Common Laboratory Accidents. *Appl. Microbiol. 16*:146-150 (1968); **Reitman, M., and A.G. Wedum:** Microbiological Safety. *Public Health Rep. 71*:659-665 (1956).

[B] Mean number of viable colonies per cubic foot of air sampled.

[C] Mean diameter of the particle.

* Reprinted with permission from "Student Manual-Testing of Class II Biological Safety Cabinets," Department of Environmental Health Sciences, Harvard School of Public Health, Boston, MA.

3.   Infectious Dose

Infectious dose is the number of organisms necessary to initiate an infection in the host. It varies with the agent, the route of exposure, the virulence of the organism, and the immune status of the host. Table III contains data showing the infectious dose for man using various organisms and different routes of exposure.

Table III. Infectious Dose for Man [A]

Disease or Agent	Dose [B]	Route of Inoculation
Scrub typhus	3	Intradermal
Q fever	10	Inhalation
Tularemia	10	Inhalation
Malaria	10	Intravenous
Syphilis	57	Intradermal
Typhoid fever	10^5	Ingestion
Cholera	10^8	Ingestion
Escherichia coli	10^8	Ingestion
Shigellosis	10^9	Ingestion
Measles	0.2 [C]	Inhalation
Venezuelan encephalitis	1 [D]	Subcutaneous
Polio virus 1	2 [E]	Ingestion

Coxsackie A21	≥18	Inhalation
Influenza A2	≥790	Inhalation

A Source: Anon., 1974.

B Dose in number of organisms

C Median infectious dose in children

D Guinea pig infective dose

E Median infectious dose

* Reprinted with permission from "Student Manual-Testing of Class II Biological Safety Cabinets," Department of Environmental Health Sciences, Harvard School of Public Health, Boston, MA.

4. Workplace Occurrences

Occupational infection can be a serious concern in certain work environments. Historically, anthrax (*Bacillus anthrasis*, aerobic GPB spore-forming bacteria) had been a major occupational hazard of industrial workers who process contaminated animal hides, hair (especially from goats), bone and bone products, and wool, in addition to veterinarians and agricultural workers who handle infected animals. Farmers and slaughterhouse workers were at risk of acquiring brucellosis (*Brucella* spp.) by handling tissues, blood, urine, vaginal discharges, and aborted fetuses of infected cattle, swine, sheep, goats, horses, and reindeer.

Today, the threat of health care workers (HCWs) acquiring hepatitis B and other bloodborne pathogens has become an issue of increasing concern. Monkey handlers are at risk of exposure to the herpes simian virus, a fatal human pathogen. Q fever is also a major concern for sheep handlers. Workers in endemic areas for valley fever (e.g., the San Joaquin and Sacramento valleys) who are exposed to dust containing spores of the fungus *Coccidioides immitis* are at risk of Valley fever infection. Bird handlers, poultry farmers, and workers in poultry processing plants are at risk of acquiring psittacosis from infected birds. Workers exposed to pigeon droppings might be exposed to the fungus *Histoplasma capsulatum*, the causative agent for histoplasmosis.

In some of the occupational infection cases, the causal factors and the responsible agents might not be readily identified. For example, it was reported in 1987 that five molecular biologists working in two adjacent laboratories at the Pasteur Institute in Paris came down with cancer.[4] They were working with tumor viruses, oncogenies, and mutagens. Although neither the exact mechanism of exposure nor the identification of an infectious agent were established, the odds of having five rare cases of bone cancer in a small cluster of 50 people within a two-year period is estimated to be 1 in 10 million.

In another unusual exposure, a lab worker received an accidental injection of a human colonic adenocarcinoma cell line.[5] Such accidental "grafting" usually does not result in significant consequences since differences in tissue type will trigger the host's defense system to reject incompatible cells. In this case, however, the patient was later diagnosed to have developed a small tumor nodule at the site of inoculation.

B. Laboratory-Acquired Infections

1. Review of the Available Information

For more than 40 years, efforts have been made to study the accidental infection of laboratory workers with pathogenic microorganisms.[6-12] During this period, several studies have clearly demonstrated that bacterial, viral, fungal, and rickettsial agents are potentially hazardous to individuals within the laboratory, and to those in surrounding areas.

In 1946, the first systematic study of the potential for laboratory-acquired viral infections was initiated by Sulkin and Pike.[10] In 1951, in conjunction with the laboratory branch of the American Public Health Association (APHA), they initiated a surveillance program to obtain additional information. This program included the development, distribution, and analysis of a questionnaire that was provided to more than 5000 laboratories, a search of the published literature, and personal communications.[11] As a result, most of the information we have on accidental infections of laboratory workers with pathogenic microorganisms has come from case reports, questionnaires, publications, and personal communication. In general, these occurrences have been in the biomedical community and took place prior to the institution of modern containment practices.

Of all the studies that have complied and analyzed information on laboratory-associated infections, the most recent by Pike contains more than 4000 cases.[9] As seen in Table IV, there were 168 deaths in the 4079 cases reported, with most of the deaths occurring from bacterial and viral infections. Table V shows the 10 most frequently reported laboratory-associated infections.

Table IV. Overt Laboratory-Associated Infections with Various Classes of Agents [A]

Agent	No. of Cases	No. of Deaths	No. of Agents Involved	No. of Cases Published
Bacteria	1704	71	37	744
Viruses	1179	55	85 [B]	915
Rickettsiae	598	25	8	381
Fungi	354	5	9	313
Chlamydiae	128	10	3	71
Parasites	116	2	17	74
Total	**4079**	**168**	**159**	**2498**

[A] Source: **Pike, R.M.:** Past and Present Hazards of Working with Infectious Agents. *Arch. Pathol. Lab. Med. 102*:333-336 (1978).

[B] Of these, 36 were arboviruses.

Table V. Ten Most Frequently Reported Laboratory-Associated Infections [*]

Infection	No. of Cases	No. of Deaths
Brucellosis	426	5
Q Fever	280	1
Hepatitis	268	3
Typhoid Fever	258	20
Tularemia	225	2
Tuberculosis	194	4
Dermatomycosis	162	0
Venezuelan Equine Encephalitis	146	1
Psittacosis	116	10
Coccidioidomycosis	93	2
Total	**2168**	**48**

[*] Source: **Pike, R.M.:** Past and Present Hazards of Working with Infectious Agents. *Arch. Pathol. Lab. Med. 102*:333-336 (1978).

Note that there is no way to accurately determine the true number of laboratory acquired infections that have actually occurred throughout the years. The primary reasons for this lack of data is there has been no requirement for reporting these infections, and it is difficult to determine whether all reported infections were indeed laboratory acquired (e.g., slow developing pulmonary tuberculosis).

2.   Modes of Exposure and Population at Risk

In a report published in 1976, Pike analyzed the results of 3921 laboratory-associated infections and found that only 703 (18%) of the infections (see Table VI) were caused by identifiable accidents.[13] The remainder resulted from unknown or unrecognized causes. The most common mechanisms of exposure identified were the result of accidents involving direct inoculation by needle and syringe, cuts or abrasions from broken glass or other sharp objects, and contact resulting from spills and sprays. Of the work-related categories analyzed (see Table VII), it was found that 59% of the infections occurred in individuals engaged in research activities.

Table VI. Number of Laboratory-Associated Infections Caused by Various Accidents *

Types of Accidents	Agents							
	Bacteria	Viruses	Rickettsiae	Fungi	Chlamydiae	Parasites	Unspecified	Total
Accident involving needle and syringe	83	43	16	12	5	16	2	177
Contact with infectious material resulting from spills, sprays, etc.	82	72	11	6	8	9	0	188
Injury with broken glass or other sharp object	75	11	4	9	0	1	12	112
Aspiration through pipet	67	20	3	0	1	1	0	92
Bite or scratch of animal or ectoparasite	41	25	9	4	0	9	7	95
Other	3	0	0	0	0	0	0	3
Not indicated	27	3	2	2	0	2	0	36
Total	**378**	**174**	**45**	**33**	**14**	**38**	**21**	**703**

* Source: **Pike, R.M.:** Laboratory-Associated Infections: Summary of 3,921 Cases. *Health Lab. Sci. 13:*105-114 (1976).

Table VII. Distribution of Cases According to Primary Purposes of Work Performed *

Work	Agents							
	Bacteria	Viruses	Rickettsiae	Fungi	Chlamydiae	Parasites	Unspecified	Total
Diagnostic	386	173	27	43	10	18	20	677
Research	829	706	455	155	85	70	7	2307
Teaching	69	15	0	18	0	4	0	106
Biologic products	35	73	18	2	5	0	1	134
Unknown	350	82	73	135	28	23	6	697
Total	**1669**	**1049**	**573**	**353**	**128**	**115**	**34**	**3921**

* Source: **Pike, R.M.:** Laboratory-Associated Infections: Summary of 3,921 Cases. *Health Lab. Sci. 13:*105-114 (1976).

The importance of these data is that working with infectious agents represents a serious occupational hazard and requires specialized control measures to prevent illness.

3. Causative Agents

Although the true incidence of laboratory-acquired illness and the precise distribution of causative agents is not known, the available data seem to indicate that in the past 50 years there has been a change in the agents responsible for laboratory-acquired infections (see Table VIII). Bacterial-associated illness, for example, has declined from 67% to 13%, and viral illness has increased from 15% to 59%.[14]

Table VIII. Laboratory-Acquired Infections: Causative Agents and Changing Trends *

Agent	Period reviewed		
	1925–1934	1945–1954	1965–1974
Bacteria	67%	40%	13%
Viruses	15%	22%	59%

Rickettsiae	6%	22%	3%
Fungi	2%	8%	20%
Other	10%	8%	6%

* Source: **Liberman, D.F., and J.G. Gordon (eds):** *Biohazards Management Handbook.* New York: Marcel Dekker, Inc., 1989.

C. Bloodborne Pathogens

1. Introduction

Bloodborne diseases of concern include hepatitis B, acquired immunodeficiency syndrome (AIDS), hepatitis C, delta hepatitis, syphilis, malaria, and infection caused by cytomegalovirus. Bloodborne pathogens may be transmitted from the infected individual to other persons when blood or other body fluids are exchanged. Among these bloodborne pathogens, hepatitis B virus (HBV) and human immunodeficiency virus (HIV) are the agents of greatest concern in the occupational environment.

The increasing number of HBV infections and HBV carriers in the United States, and the grave consequence of HIV infection, make these two agents prime candidates of concern. It is important to realize that in contrast with hazardous chemical agents in the workplace, hazardous biological agents such as bloodborne pathogens have the ability to replicate. Thus, "safe" doses of chemical and physical agents may be defined; however, there is no "safe" level of a bloodborne pathogen.

2. Hepatitis Viruses

Hepatitis means "inflammation of the liver" and is caused by various agents. There are several viral agents that have been shown to cause hepatitis, including hepatitis A, B, C, D, and E.

Hepatitis A and E: Hepatitis A, also known as "infectious hepatitis," is transmitted primarily through ingestion of fecal contaminated material and water. Hepatitis E is also transmitted via ingestion of contaminated water and probably from person to person by the fecal-oral root. Neither is a bloodborne pathogen and therefore they are not major concerns in the occupational environment.

Hepatitis B: Hepatitis B, formerly called "serum hepatitis," is caused by the hepatitis B virus (HBV). Structurally, HBV has an inner core structure containing DNA, enzymes, and proteins. One of the core proteins is the hepatitis B core antigen against which antibodies are formed on infection. The outer shell is comprised of a lipoprotein and includes the hepatitis B surface antigen, another marker of exposure. Once inside the body, this virus attacks and replicates itself in liver cells.

Hepatitis B infection does not occur uniformly throughout the United States. The disease is encountered more often in certain ethnic and racial groups, and is especially prevalent in various groups related to occupation.

The percentage of people in the United States who are hepatitis B carriers (i.e., at risk of developing chronic liver disease and capable of transmitting the disease to others) is approximately 0.2% for whites, 0.7% for blacks, and as high as 13% for foreign-born Asians.[15] In 1987, the Centers for Disease Control and Prevention (CDC) estimated the total number of HBV infections in the general U.S. population to be 300,000 per year, with approximately 75,000 (25%) of those infected developing acute hepatitis. Of the estimated total of 300,000 infected individuals, 18,000 to 30,000 (6%–10%) will become HBV carriers, at risk of developing chronic liver disease (chronic active hepatitis, cirrhosis, and primary liver cancer), and capable of transmitting the disease to others.[16]

When an individual is infected with the hepatitis B virus, two responses are produced: self-limited *acute* hepatitis B and *chronic* hepatitis B infection.[15] The most frequent response found in healthy adults is the development of self-limited *acute* hepatitis and the corresponding production of a hepatitis antibody. The production of this hepatitis antibody coincides with the destruction of liver cells containing the virus, elimination of the virus from the body, and lifetime immunity against reinfection.

Following this acute infection with HBV and corresponding production of the antibody, approximately one-third of all infected individuals will experience no symptoms, one-third will experience a mild flu-like illness (which is usually not diagnosed as hepatitis), and one-third will experience more severe symptoms such as fatigue, anorexia, nausea, dark urine, abdominal pain, fever and jaundice (yellowing of the eyes and skin). These more severe symptoms occur because the destruction of liver cells — in the body's attempt to rid itself of the infection — often leads to this clinically apparent *acute* hepatitis B.

The second type of hepatitis disease outcome, which is even more severe, is *chronic* hepatitis B infection. Approximately 6%–10% of those infected with HBV cannot eliminate the virus from their liver cells. In these cases, the hepatitis antibody is produced in the body for many years, usually for life. Those in this 6%–10% group become chronic HBV carriers and are at a high risk of developing chronic persistent hepatitis, chronic active hepatitis, cirrhosis of the liver, and primary liver cancer.

Chronic persistent hepatitis is a relatively mild, nonprogressive type of liver disease experienced by approximately 25% of these carriers (the 6%–10% group). Chronic active hepatitis is a progressive, debilitating disease that can lead to cirrhosis of the liver after 5 to 10 years (experienced by another 25% of the carriers). This condition may lead to fluid accumulation in the abdomen, esophageal bleeding, coma, or even death.

Hepatitis C: There is evidence that more than one type of viral agent is involved. Hepatitis C is parenterally transmitted. Ninety percent of all post-transfusion hepatitis has been linked to this agent(s), mostly because until recently there was no screening for this agent(s) in blood banks. Drug users and transfusion recipients are major risk groups. Between 15% and 35% of acute hepatitis cases in the United States are attributed to hepatitis C, and it also causes chronic hepatitis.

Studies have indicated that health care workers are also at increased risk of acquiring hepatitis C.[15] Although the pathways of transmission have not been vigorously demonstrated, it can be presumed that accidental exposures and environmental factors (similar to those of HBV) are important.

Hepatitis D: Hepatitis D is a defective virus that only co-infects with hepatitis B. If one has received the vaccine against hepatitis B, then hepatitis D does not pose a risk.

3. Human Immunodeficiency Virus

The human immunodeficiency virus (HIV) is the appropriately named causative agent of acquired immunodeficiency syndrome (AIDS). This disease weakens the body's immune system leaving the infected individual susceptible to many life-threatening "opportunistic" diseases and cancers that are not ordinarily fatal.

HIV is a member of a group of viruses known as the human retroviruses. Structurally, this virus has an inner core containing its genetic material (RNA) which is surrounded by a shell consisting of lipids and proteins.[17] One of the proteins produced by the virus is a reverse transcriptase enzyme. This enzyme allows the transcription of RNA to DNA and thereby allows the interaction of the viral nucleic acid with the host nucleic acid. In an active infection, the HIV invades blood cells (T-lymphocytes) that are normally used for the immune response, rendering the infected individual increasingly susceptible to opportunistic infections.

Since first described, the number of reported AIDS cases in the United States has increased dramatically. For the first 5½ years of the disease's existence (1981–1987) nearly 30,000 AIDS cases were reported to the CDC.[17] By 1989, the figure had jumped to nearly 89,000 reported cases.[18] It is interesting to note that the number of AIDS cases reported each year continues to increase; however, the rate of increase has steadily declined, except in 1987 when the case definition for AIDS was revised (resulting in an abrupt increase in reported cases).

The significance of these statistics, with respect to potential occupational exposure, is that the CDC estimates between 1 and 1.5 million persons in the United States are now infected with HIV.[15] The risk to health care workers becomes apparent, since those infected eventually require medical treatment for related and unrelated conditions.

The global outlook is even worse. The World Health Organization (WHO) estimates that 8–10 million adults and 1 million children worldwide are infected with HIV. By the year 2000, 40 million persons might be infected.[19] More than 90% of these individuals will reside in developing countries.

AIDS is primarily a disease of the body's immune system. The HIV attacks the immune system, leaving those infected vulnerable to a wide range of diseases that usually lead to death. The CDC has divided the progression of HIV infection into several stages (Groups I through IV) depending on the type of signs or symptoms of infection.[15]

Group I: When infected with HIV, many individuals show no immediate symptoms. In some cases, however, within a month after exposure the first evidence of HIV infection might appear as a mononucleosis type flu called "acute retroviral syndrome." The signs and symptoms of this illness include fever, swollen lymph glands, diarrhea, fatigue, and rash.

Group II: Typically, it takes six to 12 weeks after HIV enters the body before antibodies to the virus are detectable in blood samples. However, individual reactions vary, and this seroconversion might take eight months or even longer. As mentioned previously, the majority of cases show no symptoms for months or years after infection, which means that one of the most dangerous considerations of AIDS is that these individuals can transmit the virus to others during this period.

Group III: Some HIV-infected individuals will develop an unusual persistence of one or more of the clinical symptoms shown in Table IX. At this time, there may be no indication of abnormal function of the immune system, and in the absence of other explanations unusual persistence of two or more of these symptoms for more than three months is cause for concern. These symptoms are typical of what is known as AIDS-Related Complex (ARC).

Table IX. Clinical Symptoms of HIV-Infected Individuals

- Fatigue or listlessness
- Weight loss of 10–15 pounds or 10% of body weight
- Fever of at least 100°F
- Drenching night sweats
- Swollen lymphnodes in the neck and/or armpits in addition to the groin area
- Diarrhea

Group IV: The clinical manifestations of this "full-blown AIDS" group may vary extensively. Some of these patients may develop what is known as HIV "wasting syndrome" characterized by severe involuntary weight loss, chronic diarrhea, weakness and a long-term fever of a month or more. This last syndrome alone might result in death.

As mentioned previously, an individual with full-blown AIDS is susceptible to opportunistic infections that an individual with a normal immune system would experience only rarely; therefore, there are specific diseases that are considered indicators of AIDS. Among these are parasitic diseases such as *Pneumocystis carinii* pneumonia (the most common opportunistic infection and cause of death); fungal diseases such as candidiasis of the esophagus, trachea, bronchi or lungs; viral diseases such as cytomegalovirus infection; cancer and neoplastic diseases such as Kaposi's sarcoma; and bacterial infections such as *Mycobacterium avium* complex.

AIDS is a uniformly devastating disease. Since AIDS was first recognized and reported in 1981, more than 179,000 individuals with AIDS have been reported to public health departments in the United States. Of these, more than 113,000 (63%) were reported to have died. During this period, HIV infection has emerged as a leading cause of death in the United States among men and women 45 and younger, and children between 1 and 5.[20]

4. Who is at Risk?

From an occupational health standpoint, anyone who comes into contact with (or has the potential to come into contact with) other individuals' blood or body fluids while working, is at risk of occupational exposure to bloodborne pathogens. Health care workers are by far the largest group that fall into this "at risk" category.

The CDC defines health care workers as "persons, including students and trainees, whose activities involve contact with patients or with blood or other body fluids from patients in a health care setting."[21] There are many types of health care workers identified as being "high risk." These include, but are not limited to, those listed in Table X. Besides health care personnel, there are other non-healthcare operations that have a serious potential exposure to bloodborne pathogens for their workers. Examples of these are listed in Table XI.

Table X. Examples of "High Risk" Health Care Workers

- Physicians (e.g., surgeons and pathologists)
- Dentists (e.g., periodontists, oral surgeons, endodontists)
- Dental professionals (e.g., dental hygienists and assistants)
- Nursing professionals (e.g., intravenous therapy nurses, critical care nurses)
- Laboratory personnel (e.g., phlebotomists, blood bank technicians, medical technologists)
- Operating room personnel
- Dialysis unit personnel
- Emergency room personnel
- Laundry and housekeeping personnel
- Emergency medical technicians

Table XI. Examples of "High Risk" Non-Healthcare Workers

- Morticians' services personnel (postmortem procedures)
- Firefighters
- Law enforcement personnel
- Correctional facility personnel
- Personnel involved in infectious waste disposal
- Personnel involved in service and repair of medical equipment (e.g., biomedical technicians)

5.   Routes of Transmission of AIDS and Hepatitis B

In the discussion of how the HBV and HIV are transmitted to humans, it is most important to remember that not everyone who comes into direct contact with these viruses becomes infected. The simple analogy is that not everyone exposed to a flu virus contracts the flu. The point is that there is a difference between *exposure* (the opportunity for viral invasion) and *infection* (the virus actually enters a living cell). The question that must be answered is what *type* of exposure leads to infection.

Modes of Transmission — General Public

HBV and HIV are not transmitted by casual contact. The three generally accepted modes of transmission are as follows:[17]

a. Through parenteral (direct inoculation through the skin) injection of virus-contaminated blood or blood products. This includes blood transfusions, needle-sharing among drug users, and contact with an open wound or nonintact skin.
b. Through sexual contact in which there is exchange of infected body fluids (i.e., semen, vaginal secretions).
c. From infected mothers to their babies, including in the uterus, during the birth process, and (less likely) through breast milk.

Modes of Transmission — Workplace, Patient to Health Care Worker

In the occupational setting, blood is the single most important source of HBV and HIV infection. Both of these viruses have been transmitted in the workplace by:[16]

a. Parenteral (direct inoculation through the skin) injection, which includes contact with an open wound, contact with nonintact skin (chapped, abraded, weeping skin), and injections through the skin (needle sticks and cuts with sharp instruments).
b. Mucous membrane exposure, which includes blood or blood containing body fluid contamination of the eye or mouth.

The CDC has estimated that 12,000 health care workers whose jobs entail exposure to blood become infected with hepatitis B each year. Of these 12,000, 500 to 600 are hospitalized as a result of the infection, and 700 to 1200 of those infected become HBV carriers. Of the 12,000 hepatitis B-infected workers, approximately 250 will die (12–15 from fulminant hepatitis, 170–200 from cirrhosis, and 40–50 from liver cancer).[34] These statistics support the fact that 10% to 30% of all health care workers show serologic evidence of past or present HBV infection.

On the other hand, occupational transmission of HIV has been documented in only a few health care workers. The CDC has identified only 25 cases in which HIV infection is *directly* related to occupational exposure.[15] These 25 cases represent a diverse group of health care personnel including nurses, laboratory personnel, and a dentist. In 16 of these cases, exposure to the blood of HIV-infected individuals occurred by needle stick. Two infections are believed to have resulted from cuts with sharp, HIV-contaminated objects. In the remaining seven cases, HIV exposure occurred via mucous membrane or nonintact skin.

It is important to realize that the potential for HBV transmission is greater than the potential for HIV transmission. The risk of hepatitis B infection (for an individual who has not had prior hepatitis B vaccination) following a parenteral exposure (such as a needle stick from a hepatitis B carrier) is approximately 6%–30%.[22] The risk of infection with HIV following a needle stick exposure to blood from a patient known to be infected with HIV is approximately 0.35%.[23] This rate of transmission is considerably lower than that for HBV, probably as a result of the significantly lower concentrations of virus in the blood of HIV-infected persons and the infectivity of HIV.

In addition to blood, there are numerous other body fluids that are either known or suspected in the transmission of HBV or HIV. They include cerebrospinal fluid (CSF), synovial fluid, pleural fluid, peritoneal fluid, pericardial fluid, amniotic fluid, semen, and vaginal secretions. There are several other body substances to which the risk of HBV or HIV transmission is extremely low or nonexistent, including feces, nasal secretions, sputum, sweat, tears, urine, and vomitus *unless* they contain visible blood.[24]

Modes of Transmission — Workplace, Health Care Worker to Patient

It is also worth mentioning that not only is there documentation of HIV transmission from patient to health care worker, but in 1991 the first evidence to strongly suggest HIV transmission from health care worker to patient was discovered.[25] The CDC investigation of a Florida dentist with AIDS revealed it is likely that 3 to 5 patients were infected with HIV while receiving dental care. Neither the precise mode of HIV transmission to these patients nor the reasons for transmission to multiple patients in a single practice are known. However, the hepatitis B virus has also been transmitted to multiple patients in the practice of HBV-infected health care workers during invasive procedures.[26-28]

Most reported transmissions of HBV to clusters of patients in the United States occurred before awareness increased of the risks of transmission of bloodborne pathogens and before emphasis was placed on the use of "Universal Precautions" and hepatitis B vaccine among health care workers. Factors that may be associated with this transmission of bloodborne pathogens from infected health care worker to patients include variations in procedures performed and techniques used by the health care worker; infection control precautions used; and the titer of the infecting agent.

6. Regulatory Requirements

During the 1980s, the CDC and OSHA were involved in recommending and setting regulatory reuirements to control occupational exposure to bloodborne pathogens.

Centers for Disease Control and Prevention: In 1983, the CDC published a report titled "Guidelines for Isolation Precautions in Hospitals." One section of this document ("Blood and Body Fluid Precautions") recommended that blood and body fluid precautions be taken when a patient was known or suspected to be infected with bloodborne pathogens.

The CDC later published a report titled "Recommendations for Prevention of HIV Transmission in Health-Care Settings." This 1987 report, in contrast with the 1983 document, recommended that blood and body fluid precautions be consistently taken for *all* patients regardless of their bloodborne infection status. This extension of blood and body fluid precautions to all patients is referred to as "Universal Blood and Body Fluid Precautions" or "Universal Precautions." Under Universal Precautions, the blood and certain body fluids of all patients are considered to be potentially infectious for HIV, the hepatitis B virus, and other bloodborne pathogens.

In July of 1991, the CDC released "Recommendations for Preventing Transmission of HIV and HBV to Patients During Exposure-Prone Invasive Procedures."[29] These recommendations were developed to update the CDC's previous recommendations for prevention of HIV and HBV transmission in health care settings. According to the recommendations, as long as the health care worker adheres to appropriate infection control procedures, the risk of transmitting HBV from an infected health care worker to a patient is small, and the risk of transmitting HIV is likely to be even smaller. However, according to the recommendations, the likelihood of exposure of the patient to a health care worker's blood is greater for certain procedures designated as "exposure-prone." Thus, health care workers who perform exposure-prone procedures should know their HBV and HIV status. Health care workers who are infected with HIV or HBV should not perform exposure-prone procedures unless they notify prospective patients of their seropositivity and have sought counsel from an expert review panel and have been advised under what circumstances, if any, they may continue to perform these procedures.

The CDC recommendations do not call for mandatory testing of health care workers for HIV or HBV. The CDC believes the current assessment of the risk that health care workers will transmit HIV or HBV to patients during exposure-prone procedures does not support the diversion of resources required to implement mandatory testing programs.

Occupational Safety and Health Administration: In 1983, OSHA issued a set of voluntary guidelines designed to reduce the risk of occupational exposure to the hepatitis B virus. These guidelines were sent to health care employers throughout the United States. In November of 1987, OSHA published an "Advanced Notice of Proposed Rulemaking" announcing the initiation of the rulemaking process to develop a standard for protecting employees from HBV and HIV.

In December of 1991, OSHA issued its final standard to protect workers from bloodborne pathogens. This standard represented OSHA's first regulation of occupational exposure to biological hazards. The following is a summary of the key provisions of the final bloodborne pathogens standard as it applies to each employer having employees with occupational exposure to blood or other potentially infectious materials:[30]

Exposure Control Plan: Each employer must develop a written exposure control plan to eliminate or minimize employee exposure to bloodborne pathogens. The plan must include an exposure determination to identify potentially exposed employees. The plan should also include a schedule and method for implementing other provisions of the standard, such as hepatitis B vaccination, post-exposure evaluation and follow-up, communication of hazards to employees, and record keeping. See Appendix V — "Example of a Generic Bloodborne Pathogens Written Exposure Control Plan" — which should be used only as a guide to design a site-specific control plan.

Methods of Compliance: Engineering and work practice controls are designated as the primary means of eliminating or minimizing employee exposures. The standard defines engineering controls as "controls that isolate or remove the bloodborne pathogens hazard from the workplace." Also, Universal Precautions, which prevent contact with blood or other potentially infectious materials, are mandated by the standard.

Housekeeping: Employers must ensure that the work site is clean and sanitary. All equipment and surfaces must be cleaned and decontaminated after contact with blood or other potentially infectious materials.

Hepatitis B Vaccination: Employers must make the hepatitis B vaccination available at no cost to employees who have occupational exposure.

Communication of Hazards to Employees: Warning labels are required on all containers of regulated waste, refrigerators, and freezers containing blood or other infectious materials; and other containers used to store, transport, or ship blood or other infectious materials.

Information and Training: All employees with occupational exposure must participate in a training program provided at no charge. Training must be provided at the time of initial assignment and at least annually thereafter.

Record Keeping: Each employer must establish and maintain employee medical records that include: name; social security number; hepatitis B vaccination status; and results of examinations, tests, and follow-ups.

D. Tuberculosis

1. Introduction

Tuberculosis (TB) has been known to man for centuries. In the 18th and 19th centuries, the disease was known as the white plague. The disease was recognized in the United States as early as the mid-1700s, and as the U.S. population grew, so did the TB mortality rate. Tuberculosis, in fact, was the leading cause of death in the United States in 1900, causing approximately 10% of all deaths.[31]

In 1944, the U.S. Public Health Service Tuberculosis Program was initiated, and the annual number of TB cases declined steadily for several decades; however, the number of TB cases reported to the CDC has risen since 1988.[32] In 1990, 25,701 cases were reported, an increase of 9.4% from the 1989 figure and the largest annual increase since 1952. From 1985 to 1990, reported cases increased by 15.8%.

Tuberculosis is still a serious medical problem in many developing countries today. WHO estimates that 1.76 billion people worldwide are infected, 8 to 10 million new cases occur each year, and 2 to 3 million people die from TB each year.[33]

2. What is Tuberculosis?

Tuberculosis is an infectious disease caused by the tubercle bacillus, *Mycobacterium tuberculosis* (*M. tuberculosis*). The word "tubercle" means a nodule or small lump. Tuberculosis most commonly involves the formation of tubercles, fibrosis or inflammatory infiltrations in the respiratory system.

Diagnosis and treatment of TB is relatively simple and effective. There are four basic methods used in the diagnosing of TB:

- Detailed medical history, including previous potential exposure to TB, living arrangements, and ethnic origin;
- Tuberculin skin test, which involves the injection of purified protein derivative (PPD) onto the forearm and subsequent observation for swelling around the site of injection;
- Chest X-ray to monitor for pulmonary tuberculosis; and
- Bacteriologic exam of the patient's sputum for acid-fast bacteria.

Once an individual is diagnosed with TB, chemotherapeutic drugs such as rifampin, ethambutol, isoniazid, and para-amino-salicylic acid are used for 9 to 24 months treatment regimens. When a patient is unable to maintain his or her treatment regimen, perhaps as a result of substance abuse or homelessness, the intermittent administration of medication can result in drug resistant strains of TB.

3. Disease Transmission

M. tuberculosis is carried in airborne particles, known as droplet nuclei, generated when persons with pulmonary or laryngeal TB sneeze, cough, speak, or sing.[34] The droplet nuclei carrying the *M. tuberculosis* are generally 1–5 μm in size and are easily deposited in the gas-exchange regions of the lung. Once deposited into the lung, the *M. tuberculosis* is capable of multiplying and spreading through the lung to lymph nodes and other parts of the body.

4. Who is at Risk?

The status of the immune system is the key to a recently infected individual developing TB. A healthy person's immune system will usually contain the spread of the tubercle bacilli but will not completely eliminate them from the body. In the United States, only about 5% of newly infected individuals will develop TB within the first few years following infection. The remaining 95% usually are not even aware they have been infected.[31] In these individuals, at any time in the future if the *M. tuberculosis* overcomes the body's immune system, active TB can occur.

According to the American Medical Association (AMA), about 70% of infectious TB cases occur among racial and ethnic minorities.[35] About 10% of those infected will develop active TB at some time in their lives.

TB is not evenly distributed throughout all segments of the U.S. population. Groups known to have a high incidence include blacks, Asian and Pacific Islanders, American Indians and Alaskan Natives, Hispanics, current or past prison inmates, alcoholics, intravenous (IV) drug users, the elderly, foreign-born persons from areas of the world having a high prevalence of TB, and individuals living in the same household as members of these groups.[36]

Because the probability that a susceptible person will become infected depends largely on the concentration of infectious droplet nuclei in the air, it is obvious that social conditions such as overcrowding in homes or correctional facilities plays a large role in transmission. Also, individuals who are not healthy and have a weakened immune system will be more likely to develop the disease. In HIV-infected individuals, for example, the immune system is suppressed and will be unable to fight the spread of tubercle bacilli. The HIV-infected individual therefore is at a greater risk of developing and transmitting TB.

From an occupational health standpoint, TB transmission is widely recognized as a high risk to personnel who work in health care settings such as nursing homes and hospitals. The magnitude of risk to the health care worker varies considerably by type of health care setting, patient population served, job category, and the area of the facility in which a person works. Workers in the correctional facilities are also recognized to be at high risk.

5.   Preventing Occupational Transmission of Tuberculosis

The transmission of TB can be minimized or prevented in the workplace if a blend of appropriate control methods are effectively implemented. There are three types of control methods for minimizing TB transmission: administrative controls, engineering controls, and work practices including appropriate personal protective equipment (PPE). Each of these control methods and how they apply to the health care setting is discussed below.

Administrative Controls

Early identification (diagnosis) of patients with TB infection or active TB is critical in the health care setting. Once identified, appropriate precautions can be taken. For example, these patients can be put into patient isolation rooms with special ventilation systems that prevent the buildup or spread of droplet nuclei containing *M. tuberculosis*; therefore, hospitals with high risk patient populations should implement systems to identify these patients as quickly as possible.

Engineering Controls

As mentioned above, ventilation can be used as an effective method to control TB transmission. Both local exhaust ventilation and general dilution ventilation can be used. Continuously recirculating air in a patient room occupied by a TB-infected patient may result in an accumulation or concentration of infectious droplet nuclei. Dilution ventilation reduces this concentration of contaminants by introducing "fresh" air that does not contain the contaminants.

In patient rooms, it is recommended that air be removed from the room by exhaust directly to the outside of the building. Air supply into the patient room is then provided with air that does not contain the contaminants. In general use areas such as emergency, treatment, and waiting rooms, recirculated air is an alternative to using large percentages of fresh outside air.

If air is recirculated, care must be taken to ensure infection is not transmitted in the process. To prevent this, high-efficiency particulate air (HEPA) filters can be used. HEPA filters remove at least 99.97% of airborne particles larger than 0.3 microns in diameter; theoretically, they should remove infectious droplet nuclei.[37] Local exhaust ventilation can be used as a source control technique that removes airborne contaminants at their source. For example, the use of a booth with an exhaust fan maintaining continuous negative pressure can effectively control *M. tuberculosis* spread during sputum induction procedures.

Germicidal ultraviolet (UV) lamps can also be used to prevent TB transmission; however, their effectiveness remains controversial. UV lights can be installed into air supply ductwork as an air disinfection system or more rarely installed into work environments where employees wear proper personal protective equipment to protect them from the adverse effects of UV radiation.

<u>**Work Practices Including the Use of Personal Protective Equipment (PPE)**</u>

Specific work practices that include the wearing of various types of PPE should be used by the health care worker to prevent transmission of TB. Surgical masks, respirators, and Universal Precautions barrier equipment are effective in accomplishing this. Because TB is transmitted primarily through the air, surgical masks and respirators are most important.

Standard surgical masks provide protection as a shield against sprayed droplets generated directly from coughing and sneezing, but they generally are not as effective in preventing inhalation of droplet nuclei (floating in air) because of their inability to provide a tight seal to the face. The CDC recommends the use of disposable particulate respirators that can better filter droplet nuclei in the 1–5 micron range. Appropriate fit testing for these particulate respirators is also recommended by the CDC.

In 1992, the National Institute for Occupational Safety and Health recommended that NIOSH-certified, powered, half-mask respirators equipped with HEPA filters be used in conjunction with an effective respiratory program.[37] These powered, air-purifying respirators (PAPRs) are recommended for certain hazardous locations and procedures such as sputum induction (induced patient coughing). It is yet to be scientifically determined which of these respirators is most appropriate and effective for health care workers.

E. Sampling Methods for Viable Microorganisms

1. Introduction

Sampling methods for the collection and evaluation of biohazards parallel those methods already used in the industrial hygiene field with one primary distinction: the biohazard may be a viable organism. As is the situation when sampling for physical or chemical substances, proper evaluation of the hazard depends on minimizing sample loss between collection and evaluation stages. Nonviable materials require physical or chemical stabilization to maintain their identity for evaluation purposes. Viable organisms, however, must be collected so that the viability of the organism is sustained for evaluation purposes. The emphasis of the methods and procedures discussed below will concentrate on sampling for viable microorganisms.

Sampling methods for microorganisms can be categorized on the basis of the substrate being sampled and the purpose of the sample collection. Substrates that can be sampled include liquids, surfaces, and the air. Microbial sampling is useful for infection control, clean room verification, product quality assessment, or to assess environmental quality relative to perceived or actual health risk. The methods, procedures, and types of instrumentation indicated below will give the industrial hygienist a reference point from which to begin an investigation.

2. Sampling of Liquids and Fluids

Liquids that can be sampled for biological growth range from sewage treatment plant effluents, industrial waste water, food processing waste water, hospital and clinical laboratory wastes to cooling tower waters and industrial fluids from metal-working coolants and engine lubricating oils to industrial process waters.

In most cases, the easiest method of collecting a sample of the liquid for analysis is to obtain a representative sample in a sterilized container. Commercial devices are available for sampling from large bodies of water such as lagoons and ponds; examples are the Kemmerer sampler, the van Dorn sampler, and the Nasen bottle. These devices allow for sampling at a desired depth within the body of water. On a continuous flow system or pipe system, rubber diaphragms can be mounted from which a grab sample can be secured with a sterile syringe. Diverter valves can also be placed in-line to secure a liquid sample. Sampling protocols and descriptions of sampling devices can be found in limnology textbooks or the APHA's *Standard Methods for the Examination of Water and Wastewater*.[38]

Membrane filters can also be used for sampling fluids. This method is particularly effective for quantitation of microorganisms present at very low densities where large volumes of liquid must be sampled.[37] The filter membrane can be placed directly on a nutrient medium and incubated. If the concentration is high, the microorganisms can be eluted from the membrane, diluted in media, and placed on nutrient medium for analysis.

Recent advances in the detection of microorganisms in industrial fluids include the development of commercially available dip slides. A slide with prepared medium is dipped into the fluid, placed back in its container, incubated at an appropriate temperature for a prescribed time and the results compared to a calibration chart. Advantages of this method are: 1) it is easy to use; 2) it is accurate and semi-quantitative; and 3) it allows colonies to form directly on the slide. However, low levels ($<10^3$ CFU/mL)* of microbial contamination are not regularly detectable. One device of this type — Easicult® (manufactured by Orion Diagnostica) — has slides that will detect aerobic bacteria, contamination by yeasts and fungi, coliform bacterial growth, and a tube test that shows contamination due to anaerobic sulphide-generating bacteria.

Regardless of the type of collection device used, the sample conditions at the collection point should be maintained as closely as possible during transport of the bulk sample for analysis. Changes in environmental parameters (such as light, temperature, or relative humidity) can have a detrimental effect on the viability of the sample microorganisms. Liquid samples are the easiest type to secure and transport for analysis; however, as a general rule all microbiological samples should be analyzed as soon as possible.

3. Sampling Surfaces

Sampling of surfaces has evolved from early concerns about the spread of viral and bacterial infections from multiple-use eating utensils and the search for reservoirs of epidemic causing organisms in health care institutions to current uses such as the evaluation of laminar flow clean rooms. During the 1930s, the swab-rinse, the rinse, and the agar contact methods were developed for the measurement of contamination on utensils. These techniques were applied in other areas such as food, dairy and medical microbiology.

As new problems arose, modifications of the basic techniques were made for specific problems. The principal factors that influence the selection of a particular technique are: 1) the type and chemical composition of the surfaces; 2) the expected levels and types of contamination; and 3) the objective of the sampling test. Some tests are designed only to provide an index of sanitation; others are concerned with precise quantitation of microorganisms on surfaces.

There are five basic methods for enumerating microorganisms on surfaces: the swab-rinse; the rinse; the agar contact; direct-surface agar plating; and vacuum sampling. Several other methods described in the literature are modifications of these techniques.

Swab-Rinse Method

Early developments of this method consisted of moistening a sterile cotton swab with sterile diluent and rubbing the swab over the test surface. The top of the swab is then aseptically placed into a tube containing a sterile diluent and shaken, and the rinse fluid plated on an appropriate culture medium. Although this technique is widely used, it has several disadvantages. There is a poor correlation between the amount of microbial contamination present and that recovered by different investigators. This is partially because different types of soil or dust to which microorganisms adhere are removed at different rates depending on the chemical and physical properties of the surface and the diluent used to moisten the swab. Also, individual techniques vary with respect to speed and pressure. Elution from the cotton may be incomplete, reducing the actual count. Substitution of other types of swab materials (such as synthetic fibers) has been investigated and found to give better results than cotton wool.[39]

---

* A colony is a discrete accumulation of microbial growth on the surface of a solid culture medium which is visible to the naked eye. A colony can be the result of the growth and multiplication of a single microbial cell or of a clump of two or more cells. Colony forming unit (CFU) is a measure of the number of colonies formed.

Swabs composed of calcium alginate wool have been used for surface sampling. Alginate swabs can be dissolved in Ringer's solution or a sodium hexametaphosphate solution, thus freeing the entrapped microorganisms. There is some evidence, however, that an alginate swab is not as efficient as a cotton swab in picking up organisms[40] and that the alginate may be inhibitory to some microorganisms.[41]

In some situations, a surface can be swabbed with a moist cotton swab and then rubbed over the surface of an agar medium. This technique is used for making gross estimates of surface contaminants or detecting the presence of one type of microorganism using a selective medium.

Although the swab rinse method is simple and easy to use, because of its semiquantitative nature, it is best used as a field test that provides an estimate of contamination rather than as a precise laboratory technique for measuring surface contamination.

A modification of the swab-rinse technique uses a sterile velvet pad in place of a cotton swab. The velvet pad is of standard size and shape. After sampling by imprinting on the test surface, the pad is either imprinted onto blood agar or other suitable medium (Velvet Pad Imprint — VPI Technique) or transferred to a sterile solution for rinsing (Velvet Pad Rinse — VPR Technique). A comparison of the two methods showed the VPR technique to improve bacterial recovery by as much as a factor of 20, with both samples secured in the same manner. Also, VPR was evaluated and found to yield a constant recovery rate of bacteria of 93% when rinsed in saline solutions.[42]

Rinse Sampling

In rinse sampling, the contaminated surface is immersed in a sterile fluid that is either manually or mechanically agitated to detach microorganisms. The rinse technique is more accurate and precise than the swab method because the entire surface is sampled. This limits the sampling to small areas or objects. However, one method of sampling surface contamination levels uses stainless steel strips of known dimension which, after exposure, are placed in bottles containing a 1% sterile peptone water and subjected to ultrasonic energy or mechanical agitation. The rinse fluid is then plated on agar medium.[43]

This technique has been used primarily to measure surface contamination in spacecraft assembly areas and in laminar flow clean rooms used for the assembly and test of space hardware required to be sterilized by dry heat. The stainless steel collecting technique was shown to be a more sensitive and reliable method for assessing airborne microbial contamination in an industrial clean room than the use of volumetric air samples.[44]

There have also been studies to determine the level of microbial contamination present in hospital carpeting.[45] One method involved a modified rinse technique that consists of cutting plugs out of the carpet, placing them in sterile fluid, and eluting the contaminants with a homogenizer or ultrasound energy. Rinse sampling has been applied to culturing bacteria from hands to search for reservoirs of epidemic-causing bacteria and as a surveillance technique to evaluate general levels of cleanliness.

The most efficient method for sampling the hands involves inserting the hands to the wrist in 1-quart sterilized polyethylene bags (e.g., Ziploc® storage bags sterilized with ethylene oxide) containing a known volume of sterile sampling solution. After inserting the hand, the subject holds the bag opening around the wrist. The hand is then rubbed around the wall of the bag to agitate and dislodge the microorganisms on the hand surface. The fluid is then assayed for contamination. This method permits satisfactory quantitation and identification of surface organisms and of a variable proportion of subsurface organisms.

Agar Contact Sampling Method

There are many modifications of the agar contact technique, but most are based on the same principle. A nutrient agar is pressed against the surface to be examined, removed, and incubated. The most widely used container for this purpose is the commercially available Replicate Organism Direct Agar Contact (RODAC) plate. Sterile RODAC plates are designed so that the bottom part of the plate can be filled with agar, resulting in a raised surface of culture medium for contact with the surface to be sampled. The top part of the plate fits over the bottom part without touching the agar surface.

Dilution of the sample is not possible, limiting the method to surfaces with relatively low numbers of contaminants. The presence of molds or spreading colonies sometimes makes it difficult to obtain accurate counts. This method is most useful for sampling flat, smooth surfaces. Although accuracy is relatively low, the precision of the method is high. It is an excellent method for field studies because of its simplicity and portability.

One modification of the contact agar method uses a sterilized 20- or 50-mL syringe cut off at the needle end to expose the whole of the internal diameter.[46] The syringe is then "loaded" with agar, the agar is allowed to solidify, and as needed a suitable amount of pressure is applied to expel about half an inch of agar medium directly to the surface to be sampled. Using a sterilized knife, a disc of the culture medium is then cut off and placed in a sterile Petri dish which can be incubated without further handling.

Sterilized adhesive tape can also be used to collect surface samples. After sampling by pressing the tape to the test surface, the tape can either be stained and examined microscopically or placed in a small petri dish and covered with agar for culturing.

A more recent study reported on a method for quantitating the number of bacteria on a moist surface (e.g., body tissue) by using a membrane filter contact technique. The sterile filter is applied directly to the moist surface to be sampled. Bacteria are presumably adsorbed onto the filter and trapped in its interstitial spaces. Depending on the specific surface blotting might make it easier to recover microorganisms. The membrane filter with trapped bacteria is then placed on a nutrient medium for culture and quantitation. This method, using a 5-μm membrane filter, recovered significantly more bacteria from contaminated surfaces than the RODAC plates, velvet pads, or smaller pore membrane filters.[47]

Direct-Surface Agar Plating

Microbial contaminants on surfaces can be demonstrated on site by the direct surface agar plate method. Sterile agar medium is poured on the surface area to be sampled and left to solidify, the agar being protected from contamination by a suitable cover. After incubation, the colonies at the agar surface interface are counted. A modification involves placing a small surface in a sterile Petri dish and overlaying it with an agar medium.

As a laboratory tool, the technique is accurate in enumerating surface contaminants. Field application is limited because most surfaces of interest are fixed and difficult to incubate at proper temperatures. Also, it cannot be used on surfaces containing residual amounts of bactericidal or bacteriostatic chemicals that would inhibit the growth of microorganisms.

Under conditions of normal incubation for a given type of microorganism, colonies may coalescence when microbial contamination is high, precluding use of the method with relatively dirty surfaces.

Vacuum Probe Surface Sampling

The vacuum probe surface sampler consists of a piece of Teflon® tubing with a critical orifice connected to a conical aluminum chamber. A sterile membrane filter is located at the end of the chamber. Under vacuum, particles on the surface are removed and impinged on the filter. The filter is removed, overlaid with a nutrient medium, incubated, and bacterial colonies counted. Evaluation of this method demonstrated that the probe proved to be an effective sampling device, removing 98% and recovering 88% of the surface contamination resulting from the accumulation of airborne microorganisms.[48]

When compared directly to the swab-rinse technique, the vacuum probe recovered twice as many microorganisms. This technique is suitable for sampling larger surface areas where the level of microbial contamination is relatively low and where data from small areas cannot be reliably extrapolated, such as in laminar flow clean rooms.

All of the assay procedures described above depend on the multiplication of microorganisms to form countable colonies on a nutrient medium. For this reason, if information is required on the number of microorganisms on a surface, the bacterial clumps must be broken up for assay. On the other hand, if only the number of particles bearing viable organisms is required, a different technique must be used.

Factors that must be considered when selecting an assay procedure include the number and type of microorganisms present on the surface, the nature of the surface, and whether a bactericide is present. To complicate matters further, there is no one incubation condition for which all microorganisms will grow rapidly enough to be countable after a relatively short incubation period. No one assay procedure can completely characterize the microbial contamination on a surface. It is only when all of the factors are considered that one can judiciously select one or more techniques necessary to assess surface contamination under a specific set of assumptions.

4.   Sampling Airborne Microorganisms

Bioaerosols are airborne particles, large molecules, or volatile compounds that are living or released from a living organism.[49] There are numerous reasons for sampling airborne microorganisms. Sampling may aid in establishing the cause and mechanism by which infectious diseases are spread; identifying the potential for biological contamination and containment in the pharmaceutical, food producing, and brewing industries; and evaluating indoor air quality problems when microbials are suspected as the cause of infectious, allergenic or toxigenic disease(s). Guidelines published by ASTM and the American Conference of Governmental Industrial Hygienists (ACGIH) complement this manual.

Ideally, sampling of bioaerosols should be evaluated in the context of a continuum; each result is viewed in the context of previous results at that location. Long-term trends in numbers and change in flora can indicate subtle changes or problems for an environment and, for a given sample, unusual numbers or species might indicate more acute problems. This strategy is applied more easily in a manufacturing (e.g., biotechnology) environment than for assessment of indoor air quality. Within the manufacturing environment, "alert" or "action" levels can be established based on normal operating conditions. These levels, derived from historical data obtained in each manufacturing environment, serve as guides to implement corrective action. There are no action levels or standards for indoor air, and caution is urged when using bioaerosol sampling results as a basis for remedial action.

The limitations of sampling for bioaerosols must be understood to interpret laboratory results. Bioaerosol contamination of indoor environments may occur as discrete, discontinuous, nonhomogeneous, dynamic events. Without a well-designed sampling strategy, it is unlikely that bioaerosol sampling will adequately characterize the environment. In designing a sampling strategy the following issues should be addressed:

- The goal of air sampling must be clearly defined (e.g., outbreak investigation, periodic surveillance);
- Competent personnel must design and supervise the sampling strategy;
- Equipment must be calibrated properly and a written protocol made available for its use;
- Appropriate controls must be included in a sampling program;
- A sample site-selection strategy must be developed and justified; and
- The number and frequency of samples justified.

Even with a well-designed sampling strategy, other conditions might limit the interpretation of bioaerosol samples. First, conditions at the time of sampling may be different than when the problem occurred; second, the delay in receiving results form traditional test methods (e.g., incubation of culture plates) may no longer apply to current conditions. Furthermore, for environments with low levels of microorganisms, representative data is difficult to obtain because of limitations in the volume of air sampled and the number of samples collected. The limit of detection of the test methods must be considered when zero counts are obtained.

Presuming that a well-designed sampling strategy is in place, one must also be aware that the analytical limitations will not allow the detection of all viable microbes, including:

- media selectivity;
- colony overlap (high concentration) or antagonism;
- sampling technique;
- CFU vs. total number of reproductive units; and
- laboratory capability and quality assurance

Each of the sampling methods described have limitations and currently there is no single sampling method that will allow the complete characterization of an environment.

5.   Sampling Equipment

Bioaerosol samplers can be placed into three general categories: inertial impactors; filtration devices; and gravity samplers. Electrostatic precipitators rarely are used to collect biological agents.

Inertial Collectors

With this type of sampler, use is made of the knowledge that particles moving in an airstream have a characteristic inertia and may be deflected from their original path onto a surface, to be trapped by impaction, or when using a liquid to be trapped by impingement. The inertia of the particles depends on their size and weight, and knowledge of these facts is used to design samplers.

Settling Plates

Settling plates are the simplest form of biological sampler. They usually consist of open Petri dishes containing nutrient agar onto which particles will settle because of gravity.

Incubation of the plate will produce colonies corresponding to the biological organisms present in the aerosol or on the particles. This method is best-suited for conditions of still air since only large particles are able to overcome the buoyancy of the air medium. Smaller particles, especially those less than 3 ìm, settle very slowly and are not easily detectable by this method. The agar settling plate method can yield only qualitative information on the air in an environment, and if the number of microorganisms in a specific volume of air is to be quantified accurately the total airflow through the sampling device must be measured. Settling plates as a whole provide poor data and are not recommended for bioaerosol sampling.

Impingers

The all-glass impinger (AGI) functions essentially by bubbling air at high velocity through an isotonic collecting fluid. After collection, the fluid is diluted and portions are either plated or passed through a membrane filter, which is then placed on a suitable agar medium and incubated.

The impinger has a small jet or slit through which air is drawn, increasing the inertial velocity of particles in the air moving through it. The jet or slit acts as a limiting orifice and, provided a pressure drop greater than 41 cm of mercury is maintained across the orifice, it will operate at a constant flow rate of 12.5 liters per minute (L/min), which approximates the human respiratory rate.

By plating the sampling fluid onto different media and by suitable dilution techniques, this method can accommodate extreme ranges and variations of airborne concentrations. The glass impinger is easily cleaned and sterilized. The accuracy of the impinger in quantitating aerosol containing bacteria has been demonstrated to be lower than impaction methods in experiments in which the bacteria are largely single cell particles.[50]

When bacteria are carried as aggregates, impinger samplers tend to give higher bacterial counts due to the breakup of bacterial clusters. Also, liquid impingers demonstrate a higher variability than agar samplers because of analytical errors associated with plating out the samples. A recent study also indicates the detrimental effect of impinged bacterial cell survival on exposure to sunlight.[51]

Those studying outdoor aerosols should be aware that the use of transparent sampling devices such as the AGI will result in lower bacterial densities than those obtained with sampling devices that protect the liquid from sunlight. Sampling time of the AGI should be limited due to rapid evaporation of the sampling fluid. Also, because of its high impinger velocity, some sensitive organisms might not survive collection. If materials such as surfactants and antifoam are added to the collecting fluid, care should be taken to determine whether the microorganism being collected can survive these materials. Since fungal spores are hydrophobic, a filter may be placed between the impinger and pump to trap spores that are not collected in the fluid.

Impaction Samplers

These samplers operate on the principle of agar impaction, where the acceleration of air through one or more small openings is followed by the deposition of airborne viable particles onto a nutrient surface. The number of CFUs collected in a certain volume of air can then be determined by means of a simple colony count.

Slit Samplers

In the slit-to-agar sampler, air is pulled through a fixed slit onto the surface of a nutrient agar in a Petri dish, which is rotated at some predetermined speed so the microorganisms are distributed over the surface of the medium. Although most samplers have variable flow rate controls, a recommended rate of 28.3 L/min (1 cfm) is used most often. The agar plate rotation speed is also variable, which allows for the collection of both low or high concentrations of microorganisms (i.e., lower rotational speed and longer sample times for lower concentrations, and vice versa).

After the sample is collected, the agar plate is removed, incubated, and the colonies counted. A number of commercial varieties of slit-to-agar samplers are available. One potential advantage of a slit-to-agar sampler is that time/concentration plots can be developed giving temporal information relevant to barrier breakthrough, containment release, or equipment failure, as needed; however, no size selection is available with these samplers.

Large volume slit samplers use flow rates of about 1000 L/min. These types of samplers are useful for sampling extremely low concentrations where large volumes must be collected. Air is drawn through multiple slits and the particles are impacted on a rotating disc. Liquid is pumped onto the center of the disc. The spinning disc causes the liquid to move outward across the disc surface, forming a thin film that contains the deposited particles, which are collected at the edge of the disc. A modified sampler contains a device for the metered addition of sterile, distilled water to replace that lost due to evaporation during sampling.[52]

Depending on the temperature and relative humidity, evaporation can result in as much as a threefold concentration of the collecting fluid. This concentration effect can adversely affect the viability of aerosolized vegetative bacterial cells when certain high ionic strength-collecting fluids are used. These devices tend to show a greater collection efficiency for larger particles (> 2.3 µm). With particles of 0.5 µm, the collection efficiencies were demonstrated to be approximately 70%.[53]

Cascade Impactors

The cascade impactor is used to collect airborne particles onto microscope slides or filters. The sample is split into a series of progressively smaller particle size ranges by decreasing the size of the jet at each stage. Once the mass median size of the particles collected at each stage is known or determined, measurements of the relative amounts collected on each slide/filter gives the size distribution of the sample tested. The particles impacted onto the slides/filter can, after suitable staining, be examined directly with a microscope or washed off and plated out onto a nutrient medium for counting and identification. This latter method may select for those organisms most resistant to the effects of environmental exposure.

Sieve Samplers

The sieve sampler consists of an aluminum container that holds a petri dish. The container is fitted with a cover whose inner edge is threaded to receive a sieve plate with 340 holes of equal diameter drilled equidistant from each other over the surface of the plate. The sieve plate can be adjusted to an appropriate height above the agar plate to maximize sampling efficiency. A flow rate of 28.3 L/min is attained through use of a flowmeter or critical orifice. Because of dehydration of the agar medium, sample periods should not exceed 15–20 min. After sampling, the Petri plates are covered and incubated.

Sequential Impaction Cascade Sieve Volumetric Samplers

Most commonly known as the Andersen Sampler, the sequential impaction cascade sieve volumetric sampler (SICSVS) uses a series of sieve plates and the principle of cascade impaction to collect viable airborne microorganisms and to separate the collected particulates based on particle size, an important characteristic when one is concerned with respiratory tract penetration. Several of these devices are available commercially; however, they all work on similar principles and design. The SICSVS consists of from 1 to 6 aluminum stages. Each stage has an air inlet section that contains 200 or 400 orifices equidistant from each other. The orifices are progressively smaller from top to bottom stages and willimpact and collect progressively smaller size particles from each stage on an agar medium placed under the successive stages.

Constant airflow is provided by either a limiting orifice or flowmeter. At a flow rate of 28.3 L/min the 6-stage sampler will provide aerodynamic sizing of particles from 7.0 µm and above to 0.65 µm. Two stages of the sampler are often used to differentiate between respirable and nonrespirable particle sizes.

The sampling time may vary from 5 min to 60 min, depending on the quantity of airborne organisms present. In those environments with high levels of microorganisms, the SICSVS must be corrected for coincidence (the probability of more than one organism entering the same orifice and being counted as a single entity). This is normally done using the procedure for positive hole correction.[54] Another approach to increasing the sampling range has been to homogenize the agar and plate by serial dilution; however, this technique may affect viability.[50]

The number of viable cells per particle may be estimated by collecting duplicate samples; the cell count may be obtained by rinsing the collected material from each plate and filtering the contents. Dividing the cell count by the particle count of the duplicate sample gives the average number of viable cells per particle for each size category.[54]

Air Centrifuge Samplers

Early air centrifuge samplers were a modification of the large industrial cyclones that are used for dust removal. They remove particles from the air by centrifugal force, normally onto the inner surface of a rotating cone or onto the walls of the apparatus from which they are washed by a liquid. The liquid sample is then analyzed for viable organisms.

A more recent development (Biotest RCS, Folex-Biotest-Schleussner, Inc., Fairfield, NJ) incorporates into its operation the principles of centrifugation and agar impaction. Air is drawn toward an impeller that is housed within an open, shallow drum, and is then accelerated by centrifugal force onto the surface of a 34-cm^2 agar medium contained on a plastic strip. The strip is removed following sample collection, incubated, and microbial colonies counted.

Recovery rates using this sampling device were significantly higher than a slit-to-agar sampler in a variety of situations.[55] The small size of the culture surface, however, allows overgrowth of organisms if the RCS is used in areas where organisms are in high concentrations. Another major disadvantage is that airflow calibration is not possible.

Filters

Filtration is probably the most commonly used means for particle sampling. By varying the type of filter, its size and the length of sampling time, wide application of this technique is possible.

Inertial filtration takes place in the fibrous type filter, in which the interstitial spaces are larger than the particles and efficiency of filtration depends on contact between particles and filter fibers within the material.

Membrane-type filters retain particles by direct action when these are larger than the effective pore size of the filter material. The plastic membranes are made of a variety of synthetic materials. Depending on the type of filter used, pore sizes may range from 0.2 μm to 8 μm.

Gelatin filters have also been used for sampling airborne microorganisms. When placed on agar the gelatin dissolves, allowing the entrapped microorganisms to grow. The gelatin reduces the effects of dehydration.

The filter is placed in a filter holder, the holder attached to a pump or vacuum source, and sample air is drawn through the filter. Sample rates may vary from 5 to 50 L/min, but sample time is limited due to dehydration of vegetative cells caused by the high volume of air passing through the filter. Following the sample period, the filter is removed and assayed. Particles can be flushed from the filter, or the filter can be covered with an appropriate nutrient medium and incubated. This method is limited, due to the dehydrating effect, to sampling for spores and resistant vegetative cells. Also, the efficiency of elution from the filter may be questionable.

A recent variation of the filter technique is the "Collection of Airborne Microorganisms on Nucleopore Filter Estimation and Analysis (CAMNEA) Method."[56] This technique uses a polycarbonate filter with a smooth surface and uniform pore size that allows more efficient enumeration of microorganisms. After collection of the sample, the filter may either be rinsed and viable organisms counted or fixed in form-aldehyde and stained *in situ* with acridine orange, then counted by fluorescence microscopy. The advantage of the staining method is that both viable and nonviable organisms can be counted. Enumeration of both viable and nonviable microorganisms may be a better indicator of the biological potency of a microbiological aerosol, since viable counts — using filtration techniques — might underestimate the actual concentration due to physical forces or desiccation at the filter surface.

Electrostatic and Thermal Precipitators

Although electrostatic forces play some part in some of the mechanical sampling devices (such as the large volume sampler) in an electrostatic collector, this force is the only one used. Particles are given an electrical charge by one of many ways, and the charged particles are collected by attraction to an electrode of opposite polarity. The efficiency of thermal precipitators depends on the fact that particles acquire a thermophoretic force in a temperature gradient and can be made to deposit onto a slide for microscopic examination. This method is very efficient for the collection of submicron particles and for use with the electron microscope. This method is not recommended for the recovery of viable biological particles.

6. Choosing a Sampling System

A list of samplers often used in sampling microbial aerosols is shown in Table XII. When selecting a sampler or samplers for use in a particular situation, it is imperative that the investigator determine *a priori* the objective of sampling. This will require that a number of factors and questions are considered before beginning a sampling program. Is the sampling being designed to measure the concentration of all organisms present in the atmosphere? Are you searching for a particular organism or group of organisms? Are the concentrations likely to be high or low? Is the number of particles or the number of cells of primary importance?

Table XII. Samplers Recommended for Collecting Viable Microbiological Aerosols and Aeroallegens.*

Sampler [A]	Operation	Sampling Rate (L/min)	Recommended Sampling Time for Viable Recovery (min)	Applications and Remarks
1. Slit or slit-to-agar impactor (a,b — some models)	Impaction onto agar in a 10-cm or a 15-cm plate on a rotating surface	30–700	1–60, depending on model and sampling situation	Provides information on aerosol concentration over time. Available with a single slit or with multiple slits and variable rotation speeds. Bulky; AC operation.
2. Sieve impactors:				
a. single-stage, portable impactor (b)	Impaction onto agar in a "rodac" plate	90 or 180	0.5–5	Portable, useful for making preliminary estimates of aerosol concentrations. Flow rate is not easily checked. Approximately 40% as efficient as the slit impactor.
b. single-stage (N-6) impactor (a,c)	Impaction onto agar in a 10-m plate	28	1–30	Approximately as efficient as the slit impactor. Bulky; AC operation.
c. two-stage impactors (a,c)	See 2b above	28	1–30	See 2b above. Divides samples into respirable and nonrespirable fractions.
d. four-stage and six-stage impactors (a,c)	See 2b above	28	1–30	See 2b above. Provides information on particle size distribution.
e. personal cascade impactor (a)	Impaction onto filters or onto media in a special tray	2	≤ 60 with filters, 5–30	Eight stages available. For viable recovery, sampler is useful only in highly contaminated environments.
3. Centrifugal sampler (b)	Impaction onto agar in plastic strips	40½	0.5	Sampler is small, portable, and useful for making preliminary estimates of aerosol concentration. Flow rate is not easily checked. Does not collect particles below 3 μm efficiently.
4. Impingers:				
a. All-glass impinger/ AGI-30 (a,c)	Impingement into liquid, jet 30 mm above impaction surface	12.5	1–30	Cells on or in larger particles are broken apart. Suitable for viral particle collection.
b. All-glass impinger/ AGI-4 (a,c)	See 4a above; jet 4 mm above impaction surface	12.5	1–30	See 4a above. More vigorous impaction than 4a above.
c. Personal impinger (a)	See 4a above	1.5	5–15	See 4a above. Provides information on personal exposures. Useful in highly contaminated areas.
d. Multistage impinger (a)	See 4a above	55	1–30	Provides information on particle size distribution. Three stages with cut points of ≥7, ≥3, and ≥1 μm. Limited availability.

5. Filters:				
a. Cassette filters (a)	Filtration	1–2	5–60	Some viable loss of microorganisms due to desiccation. Samplers are easily portable, inexpensive, and can be used for personal monitoring. Useful for collecting large amounts of aeroallergens.
b. High-volume filters (a)	Filtration	140–1400	5–60	See 5a above.
6. Settling Surfaces:				
a. Open Petri dish, settling plate	Gravity settling onto agar in plates	——	≤ 240	Collection biased toward large particles.
b. Adhesive-coated surface	Gravity settling onto a coated surface (e.g., glass microscope slides)	——	≥ 1 day, depending on aerosol concentration	See 6a above. Method used to collect aeroallergens for microscopic identification, also useful for long-term collection of hardy organisms or those suitable for immunoassay.
7. Large volume sampler (LVS) (a,c)	Combination of electro-static attraction and impaction onto a fluid-covered surface	500–10,000	Unlimited with fresh or recirculated collection fluid	Cells on or in larger particles are broken apart. Useful over a wide range of aerosol concentrations. Collection efficiency is 45%–90% that of the AGI-30.
8. Cyclone scrubbers (a)	Combination of cyclone action and impaction onto a fluid-covered surface	75–1000	See 7 above	Cells on or in larger particles are broken apart. Useful over a wide range of aerosol concentrations.
9. Spore trap (a)	Impaction and settling	10	24 hr (onto a microscopic slide), 7 days (onto a rotating drum)	Widely used outdoors for collecting fungal spores and pollen grains for microscopic identification.
10. Rotating impactor	Impaction onto adhesive-coated, rotating surface	ca. 120	Continuous or intermittent	See 9 above. Collection efficiency of 70% for particles 20–50 μm.

N/A = not applicable

A Notes (letters appearing in parentheses):
    (a) Requires a vacuum pump and flow control device, which might be available from manufacturer.
    (b) Self-contained with built-in air mover. Flow rate must be checked.
    (c) Requires a vacuum pump with capacity for flow rate of 15 L/min at ≥ 41 cm Hg.

* Source: **American Conference of Governmental Industrial Hygienists:** *Air Sampling Instruments for Evaluation of Atmospheric Contaminants, 7th Edition.* Cincinnati, Ohio: ACGIH, 1989. Reprinted with permission.

If the objective is to monitor for the presence of a low concentration of organisms, a large volume sampler should be used. If expected concentrations are very low, the sampling liquid might have to be recirculated through the sampler to obtain sufficient cells for assay or detection. A multistage sampler will also give additional information on the particle size characteristics of the airborne cells, which can be of considerable value.

The use of a slit sampler can give the most useful information on time discrimination. Particle size information can be obtained best using a SICSV style sampler. These samplers collect relatively low flow rates, which might necessitate longer sample times. With care, however, these samplers can be used both as a cell and particle collector, and they can differentiate by particle size.

Although any sampling device that can efficiently remove small particles from the air can yield material for examination, the objective is to obtain quantitative recovery of cells as much as possible in the same state of viability as they exist in the environment. Sampling devices that incorporate collection into a liquid or onto a moist surface give the highest recovery efficiencies for viable organisms. The recovery of organisms from systems involving collection on dry filters, in itself an efficient collecting system, results in low recovery of viable cells.

Another important factor in planning an air sampling program is the provision of an adequate vacuum to operate the sampling equipment. Most sampling equipment needs a control device to meter the volume of air being sampled. This is accomplished best by means of a flowmeter or use of a critical orifice using a constant vacuum source.

Take care when sampling air suspected of containing microorganisms pathogenic to man or animals. Depending on the efficiency of the collection system, the effluent from the pumps may contain small numbers of viable cells. This effluent air should be passed through a satisfactory sterilizing system before being discharged.

References

1. **Brock, T.D.:** Medical Microbiology. In *Biology of Microorganisms,* 5th Ed. Englewood Cliffs, N.J.: Prentice Hall, Inc., 1988.

2. **Kenny, M.T., and F.L. Sabel:** Particle Size Distribution of *Serratia marcescens* Aerosols Created During Common Laboratory Accidents. *Appl. Microbiol. 16:*146-150 (1968).

3. **Reitman, M., and A.G. Wedum:** Microbiological Safety. *Public Health Rep. 71:*659-665 (1956).

4. **Barbels, D.:** Escape of the Cancer Genes. *New Scientist* (July 30, 1987).

5. **Gugel, E.A., and M. Sanders:** Needle Stick Transmission of Human Colonic Adenocarcinoma. *N. Engl. J. Med. 315(23):*1487 (1986).

6. **Barkley, E., and J. Richardson (eds.):** *Biosafety in Microbiological and Biomedical Laboratories* (DHHS Pub. No. (CDC) 84-8395). Atlanta, Ga.: Centers for Disease Control, 1984.

7. **Liberman, D.F.:** Occupational Hazards: Illness in the Microbiology Laboratory. *Pub. Health Lab. 37:*118-129 (1979).

8. **Pike, R.M.:** Laboratory-Associated Infections: Summary and Analysis of 3921 Cases. *Health Lab. Sci. 13(2):*105-114 (1976).

9. **Pike, R.M.:** Past and Present Hazards of Working with Infectious Agents. *Arch. Pathol. Lab. Med. 102:*333-336 (1978).

10. **Sulkin, S.E., and R.M. Pike:** Viral Infections Contracted in the Laboratory. *N. Eng. J. Med 241:*205-213 (1949).

11. **Sulkin, S.E., and R.M. Pike:** Survey of Laboratory-Acquired Infections. *J. Am. Med. Assoc. 147:*1740-1745 (1951).

12. **Wedum, A.G.:** Laboratory Safety in Research with Infectious Aerosols. *Pub. Health Rep. 78:*619-633 (1964).

13. **Pike, R.M.:** Laboratory-Associated Infections: Summary of 3,921 Cases. *Health Lab. Sci. 13:*105-114 (1976).

14. **Liberman, D.F., and J.G. Gordon (eds):** *Biohazards Management Handbook.* New York: Marcel Dekker, Inc., 1989.

15. "Proposed OSHA Rule Governing Occupational Exposure to Bloodborne Pathogens," *Federal Register 54:*23042 (30 May 1989). p. 2175.

16. **National Institute for Occupational Safety and Health:** *Guidelines for Prevention of Transmission of Human Immunodeficiency Virus and Hepatitis B Virus to Health-Care and Public Safety Workers.* Washington, D.C.: U.S. Government Printing Office, February 1989. p. 3.

17. **Brown University:** *Managing AIDS Patients: The Healthcare Professionals' Survival Guide* (Brown University STD Update). Providence, R.I.: Manisses Communications Group, 1988. p. 2.

18. **Centers for Disease Control:** Update: Acquired Immunodeficiency Syndrome — U.S. 1981–1988. *Morbidity and Mortality Weekly Report 38:*229-236 (1989).

19. **World Health Organization:** In Point of Fact (No. 74). Geneva: World Health Organization, May 1991.

20. **Centers for Disease Control:** The HIV/AIDS Epidemic: The First 10 Years. *Morbidity and Mortality Weekly Report 40:*357-369 (1991).

21. **Centers for Disease Control:** Recommendations for Prevention of HIV Transmission in Health-Care Settings. *Morbidity and Mortality Weekly Report 36:*3S (1987).

22. **Seeff, L.B., E.C. Wright, H.J. Zimmerman, et al.:** Type B Hepatitis After Needle Stick Exposure: Prevention with Hepatitis B Immune Globulin. *Ann. Intern. Med. 88:*285-293 (1978).

23. **Wormser, G.P., C.S. Rabkin, and C. Joline:** Frequency of Nosocomial Transmission of HIV Infection Among Health Care Workers. *N. Engl. J. Med. 319:*307-308 (1988).

24. **Centers for Disease Control:** Update: Universal Precautions for Prevention of Transmission of Human Immunodeficiency Virus, Hepatitis B Virus, and Other Bloodborne Pathogens in Health-Care Settings. *Morbidity and Mortality Weekly Report 37:*378 (1988).

25. **Centers for Disease Control:** Update: Transmission of HIV Infection During Invasive Dental Procedures — Florida. *Morbidity and Mortality Weekly Report 40:*377-381 (1991).

26. **Grob, P., B. Bischoff, and R. Naeff:** Cluster of Hepatitis B Transmitted by a Physician. *Lancet 2:*1218-1220 (1981).

27. **Rimland, D., W.E. Parkin, G.B. Miller, Jr., and W.D. Schnack:** Hepatitis B Outbreak Traced to an Oral Surgeon. *N. Engl. J. Med. 296:*953-958 (1977).

28. **Ahtone, J., and R.A. Goodman:** Hepatitis B and Dental Personnel: Transmission of Human Immunodeficiency Virus and Hepatitis B Virus to Patients During Exposure-Prone Invasive Procedures. *Morbidity and Mortality Weekly Report 40 (RR-8):*1-9 (1991).

29 **Centers for Disease Control:** Recommendations for Preventing Transmission of Human Immunodeficiency Virus and Hepatitis B Virus to Patients During Exposure-Prone Invasive Procedures. *Morbidity and Mortality Weekly Report 40:*1-9 (1991).

30. "Final OSHA Standard on Bloodborne Pathogens," *Federal Register 56:*235 (6 December 1991). pp. 64175-64182.

31. **Centers for Disease Control:** *Tuberculosis Medical Orientation Course.* Atlanta, Ga.: Centers for Disease Control, September 1989.

32. **Jereb, J.A., G.D. Kelly, S.W. Dooley, Jr., G.M. Cauthen, and D.E. Snider, Jr.:** Tuberculosis Morbidity in the United States: Final Data, 1990. In "CDC Surveillance Summaries, December 1991." *Morbidity and Mortality Weekly Report 40(SS-3):*23-27 (1991).

33. **Snider, D.E.:** *TB Notes, Winter 1990.* Atlanta, Ga.: Centers for Disease Control, 1991. pp. 1-2.

34. **American Thoracic Society:** Diagnostic Standards and Classification of Tuberculosis. *Am. Rev. Respir. Dis. 142:*725-735 (1990).

35. **American Medical Association:** *Report OO of the Board of Trustees (June 1992 Annual Meeting [A-92]) — Multiple-Drug Resistant Tuberculosis: A Multifaceted Problem.* Chicago: American Medical Association, 1992.

36. **Centers for Disease Control:** Screening for Tuberculosis and Tuberculosis Infection in High-Risk Populations, and the Use of Prevention Therapy for Tuberculous Infection in the United States: Recommendations of the Advisory Committee for Elimination of Tuberculosis. *Morbidity and Mortality Weekly Report 39(RR-8):*(1990).

37. **Levin, M.A., J.R. Fischer, and V.J. Cabelli:** Quantitative Large-Volume Sampling Technique. *Appl. Microbiol. 28(3):*515-517 (1974).

38. **American Public Health Association:** *Standard Methods for the Examination of Water and Wastewater,* 18th Ed. Washington, D.C.: American Public Health Association, 1992.

39. **Ellner, P.D., and C.J. Ellner:** Survival of Bacteria on Swabs. *J. Bacteriol. 91:*905-906 (1966).

40. **Angelotti, R., M.J. Fober, K.A. Busch, and K.H. Lewis:** A Comparative Evaluation of the Methods for Determining the Bacterial Contamination of Surfaces. *Fd. Res. 23:*175 (1958).

41. **Strong, D.H., M.J. Woodburn, and M.M. Mancini:** Preliminary Observations on the Effect of Sodium Alginate on Selected Non-Sporing Organisms. *Appl. Microbiol. 9:*213-218 (1961).

42. **Raahave, D.:** New Technique for Quantitative Bacteriological Sampling of Wounds by Velvet Pads: Clinical Sampling Trial. *J. Clin. Microbiol. 2(4):*277-280 (1975a).

43. **Raahave, D.:** Experimental Evaluation of the Velvet Pad Rinse Techniques as a Microbiological Sampling Methods. *Aca. Pathol. Microbiol. Scand. 83B:*416-424 (1975b).

44. **Favero, M.S., J.R. Puleo, J.H. Marshall, and G. Oxborrow:** Comparative Levels and Types of Microbial Contamination Detected in Industrial Clean Rooms. *Appl. Microbiol. 14:*539-551 (1966).

45. **Hall, L.B., and M.J. Hartnett:** Measurement of the Bacterial Contamination on Surfaces in Hospitals. *Public Health Rep. 79:*1021 (1964).

46. **MacCulloch, D., and B.M. Cornere:** A Method for Bacteriological Sampling of Surfaces by Direct Application of Culture Media. *J. Clin. Pathol. 26(12):*977-978 (1973).

47. **Craythorn, J.M., A.G. Barbour, J.M. Matsen, M.R. Britt, and R.A. Garibaldi:** Membrane Filter Contact Technique for Bacteriological Sampling of Moist Surfaces. *J. Clin. Microbiol. 12(2):*250-255 (1980).

48. **Peterson, N.J., and W.W. Bond:** Microbiological Evaluation of the Vacuum Probe Surface Sampler. *Appl. Microbiol. 18(6):*1002-1006 (1969).

49. **American Conference of Governmental Industrial Hygienists:** *Guidelines for the Assessment of Bioaerosols in the Indoor Environment.* Cincinnati, Ohio: American Conference of Governmental Industrial Hygienists, 1989.

50. **Lundholm, M.:** Comparison of Methods for Quantitative Determinations of Airborne Bacteria and Evaluation of Total Viable Counts. *Appl. Environ. Microbiol. 44:*179-183 (1982).

51. **Fedorak, P.M., and D.W.S. Westlake:** Effect of Sunlight on Bacterial Survival in Transparent Air Samplers. *Can. J. Microbiol. 24:*618-619 (1978).

52. **Notermans, S., E.H. Kampelmacher, and M. Van Schothurst:** Studies on Sampling Methods Used in the Control of Hygiene in Poultry Processing. *J. Appl. Bact. 39:*55-61 (1975).

53. **White, L.A., D.J. Hadley, D.E. Davids, and R. Naylor:** Improved Large-Volume Sampler for the Collection of Bacterial Cells for Aerosol. *Appl. Microbiol. 29(3):*335-339 (1975).

54. **Anderson, A.A.:** New Sampler for the Collection, Sizing and Enumeration of Viable Airborne Particles. *J. Bacteriol. 76:*471-484 (1958).

55. **Placencia, A.M.:** Comparison of Bacterial Recovery by Reuter Centrifugal Air Sampler and Slit-to-Agar Sampler. *Appl. Environ. Microbiol. 44(2):*512-513 (1982).

56. **Palmgren, U., G. Stroem, G. Blomquist, and P. Malmberg:** Collection of Airborne Microorganisms on Nucleopore Filters. Estimation and Analysis — CAMNEA Method. *J. Appl. Bacteriol. 61:*401-406 (1986).

3. Toxic Substances of Biological Origin

A. Biogenic Toxins

1. Overview

Biogenic toxins include all naturally occurring substances produced by plants, animals, and microorganisms that when introduced into a host in sufficient levels might adversely affect the well-being of the host. Biogenic toxins include metabolites of living organisms, degradation products of nonliving organisms, and those materials rendered toxic by the metabolic activity of microorganisms.

Such biogenic nonliving toxic material does not share the characteristic of self-replication seen for viable organisms; however, it should be noted that the pathologic effects associated with many infectious diseases arise from the generation of toxic materials by the infecting organism. Biogenic toxic materials generated as part of an active infection are not considered in this discussion.

Biogenic toxins can cause acute toxic disease in addition to long-term genotoxic and carcinogenic effects. Acute exposures may result in an intoxication or, if the host is sensitive, an immunologic response. Depending on the dose, certain substances may cause both types of response. Sensitization apparently requires exposure to relatively high concentrations of the antigen (toxin); however, after an individual has become sensitized, much lower levels of the antigen can elicit the response. The response to allergens is discussed in another chapter.

Characteristics of a toxicosis include:

- the disease is not transmissible;
- drug or antibiotic treatments have little or no effect on the disease;
- the outbreak is usually associated with a specific product; and
- examination of the suspected product might reveal signs of biogenic (e.g., microbiological) activity.

Only the fourth characteristic would distinguish a toxicosis of biogenic origin from a nonbiogenic toxicosis.

Many bacteria, fungi, and plants produce secondary metabolites that are toxic for species other than humans. For the purpose of this discussion, however, only those biogenic components shown to be toxic to humans will be considered.

Bacterial Toxins

Bacteria produce a number of metabolites shown to be toxic to man in addition to higher plants and animals. These toxins historically have been categorized as either endotoxins or exotoxins. The term "endotoxins" is used to describe cellular components of bacteria that are not released or excreted except at death (autolysis) of the organism. Also termed cell-associated toxins, endotoxins are typically found in the cell wall of Gram-negative bacteria (GNB) and have distinct chemical composition and toxic properties from bacterial exotoxins. A detailed discussion of endotoxin is included in this chapter as a representative toxin associated with occupational exposure.

"Exotoxins" are cellular products excreted from viable organisms or released when an organism disintegrates by autolysis. Occasionally, enzymes released from cells are considered exotoxins.

Properties that distinguish bacterial exotoxins from endotoxins are shown in Table XIII. A characteristic of importance to industrial hygiene is the protein nature of exotoxins. Proteinaceous materials are more easily destroyed or degraded than lipopolysaccharides; therefore, strategies for controlling exotoxins would be different from endotoxins. Exotoxins are also more tissue-specific than endotoxins.

Table XIV lists exotoxins produced by several species of bacteria and the type of action associated with those toxins.

Table XIII. Comparison of Endotoxins and Exotoxins

Characteristic	Endotoxin	Exotoxin
Composition	Lipopolysaccharide-protein complex	Protein
Source	Cell walls of Gram-negative bacteria (GNB)	Mostly from Gram-positive bacteria (GPB)
Effects on host	Nonspecific; produces fever	Generally affects specific tissues; no fever
Thermostability	Relatively heat-stable (may resist 120°C for 1 hr)	Heat-labile; most are inactivated at 60°C to 80°C
Toxoid[A] preparation for immunization possible	No	Yes

[A] modified protein toxin that is not toxic but still causes the production of antibodies.

Table XIV. Exotoxins Produced by Representative Toxigenic Bacteria Pathogenic to Man

Bacteria (Sp.)	Toxin/Disease
Clostridium	Botulism Tetanus Gas gangrene
Corynebacterium	Diphtheria
Staphylococcus	Pyogenic infections Pyogenic infections and scarlet fever
Pasteurella	Plague
Bordetella	Whooping cough
Shigella	Dysentery

Algal Toxins

Blooms of blue-green algae (procaryotic photosynthesizing bacteria) have been documented world-wide. These blooms indicate nutrient input into fresh water systems, usually from the introduction of agricultural runoff or raw sewage. Although the impact of these blooms has focused on water quality concerns, there have been reports of rashes and blisters of the skin, lips, and genitals in swimmers exposed to toxic metabolites released from the cell or those contained in the whole cell. Blue-green algal toxins are categorized as water soluble, temperature stable peptides. A variety of types have been described from different species, including neurotoxins, hepatotoxins, and cytotoxins.

Toxins from eucaryotic species of algae are reported to be poisonous to fish, waterfowl, mussels, and clams — and subsequently to consumers (including humans) of these products. Saxitoxin, a neurotoxin produced by the red tide algae (dinoflagellates), is associated with a disorder called paralytic shellfish poisoning (PSP). PSP is considered a risk from consumption of shellfish harvested from contaminated waters. However, toxic metabolites from both the blue-green algae and the higher algal species are not typically associated with occupational exposure.

Fungal Toxins

Within the broad group of organisms called fungi, which include both aquatic and terrestrial species, only the terrestrial filamentous microfungi produce mycotoxins. The single-celled fungi called yeast do not produce mycotoxins. Although the hazards associated with eating poisonous mushrooms dates to prehistory, only recently have the hazards associated with certain filamentous fungi been recognized. Filamentous fungi may act as free living saprophytes or plant pathogens. There are several hundred different structural types of mycotoxins, and each of these may have up to 20 naturally occurring, closely related derivatives.

Mycotoxins are low-molecular weight compounds found in a wide array of edible commodities, including beans, cereals, coconuts, milk, peanuts, sweet potatoes, and commercially prepared animal feeds. The two considered to be the "most important," however, are the aflatoxins and trichothecenes. These toxins are produced by two species of *Aspergillus* (*A. flavus* and *A. parasiticus*) and selected species of *Fusarium*. Besides their toxic effects, aflatoxins have been found to have carcinogenic properties.

Aflatoxins have been shown to be highly carcinogenic for a variety of species, and epidemiologic studies suggest an association between aflatoxin consumption and liver cancer.[1] It was further demonstrated that men are more sensitive than women.[2] In addition to being a potential carcinogen, aflatoxins are also acute toxins. Outbreaks of epidemic jaundice involving severe liver disease and death have been reported in developing countries after consumption of contaminated grain products.

In the United States, acute liver toxicity was observed in animals fed grain contaminated with aflatoxin, and though there has been no association with human toxicity, the potential for intoxication exists in selected occupational environments. Two groups may be involved with occupational exposure: those handling bulk agricultural commodities such as peanuts, cereals, and animal feeds, and those involved in laboratory studies and analysis of aflatoxin. Studies suggest that exposures to aerosols of aflatoxin might be related to bronchial carcinoma, colon cancer, and liver cancer.[3]

The trichothecenes were associated with outbreaks of alimentary toxic aleukia from the consumption of badly contaminated cereals in the former Soviet Union. At higher doses the toxin damages the bone marrow and hematopoietic system and may be immunosuppressive, leading to an increased susceptibility to secondary infections. These mycotoxins are produced primarily by *Fusarium* spp. and have accounted for the "yellow rain."

Toxigenic fungi are prolific and widespread in the air and soil throughout the world. Consequently many field crops, stored products, and agricultural commodities may be contaminated. Occupational exposures may occur in these environments. Most mycotoxins are not chemically labile, and many are heat stable up to their melting points. Both physical and chemical methods of decontamination have been evaluated; some are currently being used to decontaminate agricultural commodities.

Plant Toxins

Some plants produce materials (secondary metabolites) that are resistant to plant pathogens. These secondary metabolites, of which more than 10,000 have been identified, are produced in specific tissues of healthy plants and belong to various chemical groups, including cinnamic acids, flavonoids, terpenoids, alkaloids, cyanohydrins, quinones, saponins, unsaturated lactones, benzoxazinones, allyl sulfides, thiocyanates, and polyacetylenes.

Many of these secondary metabolites have demonstrated toxicity for man. The lectins, for example, are among the most toxic substances known. Lectins are a class of proteins that bind to carbohydrates; in this capacity, they agglutinate cells or precipitate polysaccharides and glycoproteins. Lectins are polyvalent with at least two carbohydrate binding sites to allow cross-linking between cells.

Although the agglutination precipitation properties are similar to antibodies, lectins are different in several aspects. They are found in plants, microorganisms, and viruses that do not synthesize immunoglobulins. They are structurally diverse, varying in molecular size, amino acid composition, metal requirements, and three-dimensional structure. Though similar to enzymes, they are devoid of catalytic activity. More recognizable plant toxins include those from the genus *Rhus*, which includes poison oak and ivy.

Animal Toxins

Various toxins are produced by higher species of animals. These toxins are typically associated with bites and stings. Workers involved in outdoor jobs are at greatest risk.

2. Routes of Exposure

As with nonbiogenic toxins the primary route of exposure to biogenic toxin is by inhalation. Unlike infectious agents or biogenic antigens, however, there is no amplification involved in the response to biogenic toxins. In a susceptible host the amplification (reproduction) of infectious agents or the amplification of the response to an antigen (antibody formation) can result in disease. In this aspect, biogenic toxins do not differ from nonbiogenic toxins. Biogenic toxins do differ from nonbiogenic toxins in that the growth of organisms that produce the toxin cannot be predicted.

A major consideration for measuring biogenic toxins is selection of the analytical method. Toxic-specific analysis or an appropriate surrogate must be identified to adequately assess the environment in question. The same equipment used for collecting and assaying airborne dust and chemicals can be used to collect airborne biogenic toxins.

Dermal exposure is also a route of exposure for biogenic toxins. The response to the toxin may be a localized inflammatory response, such as one associated withmany plant toxins/allergens. A systemic response through percutaneous penetration also is possible.

The third major route of exposure for biogenic toxins is ingestion. Fermentation has been a valuable process in the production and preparation of different foods; however, the same characteristics that make foodstuffs a substrate for beneficial activity of nonpathogenic organisms make it a substrate for toxigenic organisms. Various organisms are associated with food intoxications, the most notable being "the church picnic" (*Staphylococcus* sp. and *Salmonella* sp.) and botulism (*Clostridium botulinum*).

3. Workplace Occurrences

Workplace exposure to biogenic toxins can occur in any indoor environment where there is extensive growth of microorganisms — either deliberately or from contamination — or from outdoor jobs that place workers in direct contact with plants, animals, or their products. Specific occupations at risk include agricultural workers (both production and processing personnel); industries based on plant or animal products (e.g., poultry processing or the natural fiber textile industry); industries based on generation of products from microorganisms (biotechnology and fermentation); office workers in environments with indoor air contaminated by either fungi or bacteria; and outdoor jobs such as road maintenance workers and migrant agricultural workers.

B. Endotoxin

1. Overview

Endotoxin makes up part of the cell envelope of Gram-negative bacteria. Since first implicated in occupational disease in 1942,[4] exposure to endotoxin has been demonstrated in a variety of work environments. Agricultural workers and processors of vegetable fiber dust seem to be at greatest risk. Levels of endotoxin in excess of 50 ng/m^3 have been reported in swine confinement buildings,[5] grain storage facilities,[6] poultry houses,[7] cotton mills,[8] and flax mills.[8] Other environments with risk include wood chip processing and saw mills; animal handling facilities; vegetable fiber and grain handling and processing; sewage treatment; humidified office buildings; and machining operations using natural and synthetic cutting fluids.

Recent studies proposed thresholds for acute pulmonary toxicity in a range of 10–33 ng/m^3 and recommended that consideration be given to limiting exposure to airborne endotoxin in work environments.[9] This recommendation was based on results demonstrating that measurement of airborne endotoxin was a more reliable predictor of the acute airways response to cotton dust than measuring gravimetric dust.

2. Physicochemical Characteristics

A molecule of endotoxin consists of three components: a polysaccharide chain, a core polysaccharide, and a lipid moiety called "Lipid A." The polysaccharide chain gives serological specificity to GNB as the "O Antigen" and is highly variable between different species of GNB. Most, if not all, of the toxicity associated with endotoxins is associated with Lipid A.[10]

The term "endotoxin" is often used interchangeably with lipopolysaccharide (LPS). They are not synonymous, however. LPS refers to the purified Lipid A and core-polysaccharide chain. Endotoxin refers to the LPS plus various other cell wall constituents (e.g., Lipid A associated protein). The material described as endotoxin more accurately reflects what occurs in the work environment. The differences in the biological activity of endotoxin and LPS are in the bioavailability of the Lipid A and enhancement of the activity of Lipid A by various cell wall constituents.[11,12]

Although Lipid A is a relatively constant factor with established toxic properties, endotoxin is a highly variable material with no consistency in its molecular arrangement in the environment. Herein lies one of the problems of relating endotoxin to specific occupational diseases.

The biological activity of endotoxin does not depend on bacterial viability. The molecule is active as a cell wall fragment, a molecular aggregate, or as part of the intact cell wall of viable or dead bacteria. Traditional methods of sterilizing materials contaminated with microbes are inadequate for destroying endotoxin. The method recommended for inactivation of endotoxin in the U.S. Pharmacopoeia (USP) is dry heat treatment at 160°C–170°C for 2 to 4 hr. This treatment removes 99%–99.9% of the activity.

Other methods of inactivation include ethylene oxide and irradiation treatment. Ethylene oxide in the presence of 50% humidity removed greater than 90% of the *Limulus* amoebocyte lysate (LAL) and pyrogenic activity; however, the treatment was not equally effective for all endotoxin preparations tested, and it was ineffective at lower levels of humidity.[13] Inactivation with Cobalt 60 at 4.7 mrads destroyed 90% of the LAL activity. Endotoxin is a refractory molecule that maintains its activity for a broad range of environmental and occupational conditions.

3. Biological Activities

Endotoxins have a wide range of biological activities involving inflammatory, hemodynamic, and immunological responses. Of most importance to occupational exposures are the activities of endotoxin in the lung. Aerosols of dust containing bacteria and bacterial fragments, as might be found in occupational dust, are of a size that can reach and be deposited at all levels of the respiratory tree.[14] Whole bacteria have particle sizes of 1–3 µm, and fragments of GNB range down to molecular aggregates. Endotoxins associated with particles deposited in the trachea and large bronchi have only a minimal biological effect because they are eliminated by mucociliary transport. However, in the distal lung, the small bronchi, the bronchioles, and the alveoli, endotoxins can have substantial biological activity. The first cell to respond to endotoxins in the distal lung is the alveolar macrophage. Endotoxin can activate the macrophage, causing the cell to produce a host of cell-derived mediators.[14] These chemical mediators can in turn interact with and cross the air-blood barrier where they recruit blood cells, polymorphonuclear neutrophilic leukocytes (PMNs), and platelets, to the interstitium and stimulate resident cells of the airways (such as mast cells) to release additional cellular mediators — resulting in a secondary amplification of the response.

Clearly, endotoxin can have a major impact on the biology of the lung. At background levels of exposure, the described responses protect the host by inactivating the endotoxin and responding physiologically to handle the insult. Repeated exposure to levels of endotoxin not ordinarily encountered, however, may overwhelm the body's capacity to effectively detoxify or eliminate the endotoxin and result in a clinical response.

Little is known clinically about the response to inhaled endotoxins. Exposure of naive subjects to airborne endotoxin can result in acute fever, dyspnea, coughing, and small reductions in FEV_1 (the forced expiratory volume of air forcibly exhaled in the first second after a maximum inspiration).[14] These symptoms parallel those found in workers or naive subjects exposed to cotton dust for the first time. This initial response in the cotton textile worker is called "mill fever." On repeated exposure, the symptoms become progressively milder and eventually disappear. They may reoccur if a worker is absent for a prolonged period and then re-exposed.

Similar acute symptoms were documented in other environments, including humidified office buildings,[15] selected agricultural environments,[16] and vegetable fiber-processing other than cotton.[14] Nevertheless, definitive studies relating symptoms in these environments to exposure to endotoxin are lacking.

The effects of repeated exposure to aerosols of endotoxins in humans are not known. Pathological evaluation of the lungs of cotton textile workers exposed to high levels of endotoxin suggests that chronic bronchitis, as characterized by goblet and bronchial cell hypertrophy, is the endpoint of exposure to cotton dust and therefore possibly endotoxin.[17] No chronic exposure studies to aerosols of pure endotoxins have been done, however.

One other area of clinical concern regarding exposure to endotoxin is the development of hyperreactive airways. Bake et al. found that aerosols of endotoxin increased bronchial hyperreactivity in naive subjects.[18] Such increases in hyperreactivity have been demonstrated in workers[19] and naive subjects[20] exposed to cotton dust. Increased bronchial hyperreactivity may enhance the susceptibility of workers to other toxic exposures; however, the role of this response in the pathogenicity of exposure to aerosols of endotoxin is not known.

4. Measurement of Endotoxin

Before development of the *Limulus* amebocyte lysate test, the method for measuring endotoxin was the rabbit pyrogenic test. Rabbits were injected with endotoxins and the increase in body temperature measured. Although the test was sensitive (100 pg range), it was not possible to establish guidelines to maintain a consistent sensitivity, primarily because of variability in the rabbit and endotoxin preparations.

In 1956, the effects of a bacterial infection in the horseshoe crab (*Limulus fen*) were described; both living and heat-treated preparations of GNB caused intravascular coagulation and death of the crab.[21] The reaction was specific for GNB. Further studies in 1963 observed that the cell-free plasma of *Limulus* blood would not coagulate in the presence of endotoxin, but in the presence of cells called amebocytes the blood coagulated.[22] These studies concluded that the coagulation system was in the amebocytes and the rate of gelation depended on the endotoxin concentration.

Figure 1 illustrates the basis of the LAL test. Amebocytes from the horseshoe crab are collected and a lysate (LAL) prepared that contains the coagulation system. On exposure to endotoxin, an enzyme cascade is activated, which results in the clotting. There is a direct relationship between the concentration of endotoxin and the rate of gelation, and either the endpoint (gelation) or rate of increase in turbidity has been used for the basis of the test. The sensitivity of the gel-clot assay is approximately 10 pg/mL. This compares with a sensitivity in the rabbit test of 100 pg/mL.

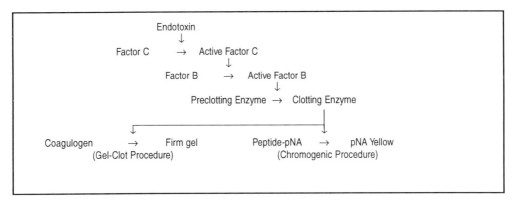

Figure 1. Clotting Mechanism of LAL Procedure.

To perform the gel-clot test, samples or a control standard endotoxin are diluted with pyrogen-free water or saline and mixed with the LAL. The preparation is incubated for a set period (usually 60 min) and the gel read by inverting the tube. A positive test is indicated by a firm gel and the endpoint is determined by comparison to a standard endotoxin.

A second assay based on clotting is the turbidimetric kinetic LAL assay, a modified turbidimetric procedure that is quantitative over a continuous range.[23] In this assay, the LAL reagent is mixed with the sample or standard and the light transmission measured at 670 nm. The turbidity is a result of formation of a visible, insoluble floc of coagulogen. At a constant time, the turbidity itself or its rate of development can be measured. Advantages of this method over the gel-clot procedure include quantification over a continuous range and some increased sensitivity, but it is no more reliable than the gel-clot method.

The third method for measuring endotoxin is the chromogenic assay. This assay is based on the cleavage of a chromophore from a synthetic peptide substrate by the clotting enzyme of LAL.[24] The activated LAL enzyme is specific for the chromophore-peptide bond. The intensity of the yellow color of the free chromophore (405 nm) is related directly to the amount of enzyme activated by the endotoxin. This method offers several advantages over the gel-clot procedure. It is faster and more sensitive by at least tenfold, it quantifies over a continuous range, and it is relatively simple. It is more expensive than the gel-clot method, however, and may be subject to more interferences — a problem that may occur frequently with environmental or occupational samples. For routine analyses, the chromogenic method might not offer any advantage over the gel-clot procedure.

Before 1982, endotoxin measurements were reported in units of weight/volume (e.g., ng/mL or ng/m³) or weight/weight (ng/mg). On June 1, 1982, the U.S. Food and Drug Administration (Center for Drugs and Biologics) began to require all manufacturers to label LAL preparations in Endotoxin Units (EUs). At that time, 1 EU was defined as 0.2 ng of the U.S. Reference Standard Endotoxin (RSE), EC-2; therefore, the conversion between ng and EU was a factor of 5 (0.2 ng/mL = 1 EU/mL). A second RSE, EC-5, has replaced EC-2 and the conversion factor is approximately 10 EU/ng. This has led to some confusion regarding the use of EUs, because different LALs have different sensitivities. Each LAL manufacturer must label the sensitivity relative to a reference standard endotoxin (RSE-2 or RSE-5).

In doing endotoxin analysis, each laboratory must confirm the sensitivity of the LAL from the manufacturer, otherwise the LAL may be contaminated.[25] The rationale for using EUs was to provide a uniform basis for comparison of results between laboratories relative to a standard. Although the concept has met limited success, much remains to be done to ensure that results between laboratories are comparable.

Much of the effort devoted to developing an assay for endotoxin has come from the need of the pharmaceutical industry to ensure that drugs are free from pyrogenic agents. The LAL procedure meets these needs. The correlation between pyrogenicity and LAL activity is good and the assay is sensitive to the picogram range.

Nevertheless, the assay does have some drawbacks that may impact its use for occupational and environmental samples. First, the LAL assay is itself a measure of biological activity, and because endotoxins act on a variety of biological systems the LAL activity might not relate to other responses caused by endotoxin. Second, the response of the *Limulus* assay varies with the molecular state of endotoxin; therefore, comparison between different environments or laboratories is difficult even when sampling and measurement parameters are carefully controlled. Third, the *Limulus* assay is subject to interferences that result in both false-positives and false-negatives. For example, polymeric molecules such as cellulose have been shown to interfere with the assay.[26] These interferences will probably occur more frequently in environmental samples. Still, the LAL procedure is the most sensitive and reliable assay available to measure endotoxin when used within the limits of the assay.

5. Environmental Sampling of Endotoxin

The collection, extraction, and analysis of aerosols for endotoxin is a relatively recent effort. In 1978, the OSHA cotton dust standard specified the vertical elutiator (VE) for measuring airborne respirable dust. Efforts to define the etiology of byssinosis resulted in the analysis of VE dust filters for endotoxin. This method has been used extensively for collecting respirable dust samples for endotoxin analysis. The filter can be weighed for a gravimetric assessment and then extracted with pyrogen-free water (containing a surfactant to facilitate extraction) and assayed by the LAL.[27] Levels of endotoxins in different environments as measured by the VE were reported by Rylander and Morey.[8]

Other methods of sampling for aerosols of endotoxin have included total dust samplers, cascade impactors, and personal samplers with separators.[5-7] Both cellulose and polyvinyl chloride filters have been used in these studies. Data have shown that the smaller size dust fractions contain greater amounts of endotoxin per unit weight of dust (ng/mg). Since endotoxins act primarily in the broncho-alveolar region of the lung, any sampling technique should provide for the separate collection of respirable particulates. All-glass impingers can also be used to sample aerosols of endotoxin; however, the stability of endotoxins in the different collection media has not been documented.

Samples of bulk materials, solid or liquid, can be evaluated using standard quantitative methodology. Extraction efficiencies for solid samples must be determined, as must stability of the extracted sample.

There currently are no established guidelines for sampling and analysis of aerosols or bulk samples for endotoxins in occupational environments. Such guidelines are necessary if comparisons between environments or laboratories can be made. Methods that are acceptable for collecting gravimetric samples of respirable dust seem to be acceptable for sampling aerosols of endotoxins. Collection of respirable particles is necessary because of the biological activity of endotoxin in the distal lung and the higher relative concentration of endotoxin on respirable particles. All materials for sample collection and analysis must be rendered free of endotoxin using documented procedures.

There also are no guidelines for the selection of filter type, and extraction efficiency studies are needed to define the optimum collection media and recovery parameters. Filters for sampling should be handled so to avoid human contamination both before and after sample collection. The appropriate storage conditions prior to sample extraction have not been defined; however, both bulk and filter samples should be stored at conditions (low moisture and temperature) to avoid bacterial growth prior to analysis. Until a simple reliable assay for endotoxin is developed, it is recommended that analysis be done by laboratories experienced in the LAL procedure.

References

1. **Stoloff, L.:** Aflatoxins — An Overview. In *Mycotoxins in Human and Animal Health* (edited by J.V. Rodricks, C.W. Hesseltine, and M.A. Mehlmann). Pard Forest South, Ill.: Pathotox Publishers, Inc., 1977. pp. 7-29.

2. **Peers, F.G., and C. Lindsel:** Dietary Aflatoxins and Human Primary Liver Cancer. *Ann. Nutr. Aliment. 31:*105-1018 (1977).

3. **Shotwell, O.L., and W.R. Burg:** Aflatoxin in Corn: Potential Hazard to Agricultural Workers. In "Agricultural Respiratory Hazards" (edited by W.D. Kelly). *Annals Am. Conf. Gov. Ind. Hyg. 2:*69-86 (June 1982).

4. **Neal, P.A., R. Schneiter, and B.H. Caminita:** Report on Acute Illness Among Rural Mattress Makers Using Low Grade, Stained Cotton. *JAMA 119:*1074-1082 (1942).

5. **Attwood, P.R., P. Brouwer, P. Ruigewaard, P. Versloot, R. DeWit, D. Heederik, and J. Boleij:** A Study of the Relationship Between Airborne Contaminants and Environmental Factors in Dutch Swine Confinement Buildings. *Am. Ind. Hyg. Assoc. J. 48(8):*745-752 (1987).

6. **DeLucca, A.J., and M.S. Palmgren:** Seasonal Variation in Aerobic Bacterial Populations and Endotoxin Concentration in Grain Dust. *Am. Ind. Hyg. Assoc. J. 48(2):*106-110 (1987).

7. **Jones, W., K. Manning, S.A. Olenchock, T. Williams, and J. Hickey:** Environmental Study of Poultry Confinement Buildings. *Am. Ind. Hyg. Assoc. J. 45(11):*760-766 (1984).

8. **Rylander, R., and P. Morey:** Airborne Endotoxin in Industries Processing Vegetable Fibers. *Am. Ind. Hyg. Assoc. J. 43:*811-812 (1983).

9. **Castellan, R.M., S.A. Olenchock, K.B. Kinsley, and J.L. Hankinson:** Inhaled Endotoxin and Decreased Spirometric Values, An Exposure-Response Relation for Cotton Dust. *N. Engl. J. Med. 317:*605-610 (1987).

10. **Galanos, C., M.A. Freudenberg, O. Luderitz, E.T. Rietschel, and O. Westphal:** Chemical, Physicochemical and Biological Properties of Bacterial Lipopolysaccharide. In *Biomedical Applications of the Horseshoe Crab (Limulidae).* New York: Alan R. Liss, Inc., 1979. pp. 321-332

11. **Helander, I., A. Salkino-Saloner, and R. Rylander:** Chemical Structure and Inhalation Toxicity of Lipopolysaccharides from Bacteria on Cotton. *Infect. Immun. 29:*859-862 (1980).

12. **Baseler, M.W., B. Fogelmark, and R. Burnell:** Differential Toxicity of Inhaled Gram-Negative Bacteria. *Infect. Immun. 40:*133-138 (1983).

13. **Tsuji, K., and S.J. Harrison:** Lumulus Amoebocyte Lysate — A Means to Monitor Inactivation of Lipopolysaccharide. In *Biomedical Applications of the Horseshoe Crab (Limulidae).* New York: Alan R. Liss, Inc., 1979. pp. 367-378.

14. **Rylander, R., and M.-C. Snella:** Endotoxins and the Lung: Cellular Reactions and Risk for Disease. *Prog. Allergy 33:*332-344 (1983).

15. **Rylander, R., P. Haglind, M. Lundholm, I. Mattsby, and K. Stenqvist:** Humidifier Fever and Endotoxin Exposure. *Clinical Allergy 8:*511-516 (1978).

16. **Rylander, R.:** Lung Diseases Caused by Organic Dust in the Farm Environment. *Am. J. Ind. Med. 103:*221-222 (1986).

17. **Pratt, C.P.:** Comparative Prevalence and Severity of Emphysema and Bronchitis at Autopsy in Cotton Mill Workers vs. Controls. *Chest 79:*49S-53S (1981).

18. **Bake, B., R. Rylander, and J. Fischer:** Airway Hyperreactivity and Bronchoconstriction after Inhalation of Cell-Bound Endotoxin. In *Proceedings of the Eleventh Cotton Dust Research Conference, Dallas, Texas* (edited by R.R. Jacobs and P.J. Wakelyn). Memphis, Tenn.: National Cotton Council, 1987. pp. 12-14

19. **Haglind, P., B. Bake, and L. Belin:** Is Mild Byssinosis Associated with Small Airways Disease? *Eur. J. Respir. Dis. 64:*449-459 (1983).

20. **Boehlecke, B., R. Schreiber, and J. Warrenfelt:** "Nonspecific Airway Reactivity Increased by Exposure to Cotton Dust." Presented at the Third International Conference on Environmental Lung Disease, Montreal, Canada, Oct. 15-18, 1986.

21. **Bang, F.B.:** A Bacterial Disease of *Limulus Polyphemus. Bull. Johns Hopkins Hosp. 98:*325-351 (1956).

22. **Levin, J., and F.B. Bang:** The Role of Endotoxin in the Extracellular Coagulation of Limulus Blood. *Bull. Johns Hopkins Hosp. 115:*265-274 (1964).

23. **Novitsky, T.J., S.S. Ryther, M.J. Case, and S.W. Watson:** Automated LAL Testing of Parenteral Drugs in the Abbot MS-2 Journal. *Parenteral Science and Technology 36:*11-16 (January/February 1982).

24. **Nachum, R., and R.N. Berdofsky:** Chronogenic Limulus Lysate Assay for Rapid Detection of Gram Negative Bacteria. *J. Clin. Microbiol. 21:*759-763 (1985).

25. **U.S. Pharmacopeial Convention:** *Bacterial Endotoxins Test, United States Pharmacopeia XXI.* Rockville, Md.: U.S. Pharmacopeial Convention, Inc., 1985. pp. 1165-1167.

26. **Pearson, F.C., J. Bohan, W. Lee, G. Brusger, M. Sagora, R. Dowe, G. Jakubowski, D. Morrison, and C. Pinarello:** Comparison of Chemical Analysis of Hollow-Fiber Dialyzer Extracts. *Artificial Organs 8:*291-298 (1984).

27. **Rylander, R., R. Burrell, and Y. Peterson (eds.):** Proceeding of Endotoxin Inhalation Workshop, Clearwater, Florida. In *The Twelfth Cotton Dust Research Conference* (edited by R.R. Jacobs and P.J. Wakelyn). Memphis, Tenn.: National Cotton Council, 1988. pp. 182-206.

4. Biogenic Allergens

A. Overview of the Immune System

Biogenic allergens include substances produced or derived from plants, animals, or microorganisms that when introduced into a host can elicit an immune response. To help in understanding the response to biogenic allergens, an overview of the immune system follows.

The primary function of the immune system is to protect the body from foreign substances by an acquired ability to distinguish self from non-self. This ability is further characterized by specificity and memory. Specificity refers to the ability to respond uniquely to many different foreign substances (antigens); memory refers to the heightened response that occurs on subsequent exposure to extremely small quantities of the original antigen.

The immune system is divided into humoral and cell-mediated components. The major cells of humoral immunity are the B-cells (B-lymphocytes). These are white blood cells that secrete proteins called antibodies which attach to foreign substances (including microorganisms) and enhance their elimination or destruction from the host. The major cells of cell-mediated immunity (CMI) are the T-lymphocytes. These are white blood cells that attack foreign substances directly.

B-cells are generated in the bursa in birds or bursal equivalent in mammals, and T-cells are generated in the thymus. T-cells can be further divided into four subsets — helper, cytotoxic, suppressor, delayed hypersensitivity — each with a specific function that modulates the immune response.

Other cell-types of importance in the immune system include natural killer cells and macrophage, both of which modulate the immune response.

1. Humoral Immunity

Humoral immunity describes the production of specific proteins (immunoglobins) by plasma cells (committed B-cells) in response to a specific antigen. There are five categories of immunoglobins (Ig) or antibodies produced by committed B-cells: IgA, IgG, IgE, IgD, and IgM. The type of biological activity elicited by a specific antigen depends on the type of antibody formed and the target cell or plasma component of the antigen-antibody complex.

On first exposure, an antigen interacts with a macrophage or other antigen-processing cell (APC), causing the release of a cellular hormones or cytokines (e.g., interleukin-1) that activate both B-cells and T-helper cells. The activated T-helper cells release other cytokines (B-cell differentiation factor and B-cell growth factor) that stimulate the proliferation and maturation of B-cells into plasma cells, which produce specific antibodies against the antigen, and sensitized B-cells, which serve as memory cells.

On second exposure, the memory cells allow a rapid antibody response to low levels of the specific antigen. The first and second antibody responses to antigen differ in their kinetics and type of antibody formed due to the previous exposure to the antigen (i.e., memory).

2. Cell-Mediated Immunity (CMI)

Cell-mediated immunity is characterized by a reaction between an antigen and a sensitized T-lymphocyte that results in an immune response based on the release of cytokines from activated cells. There is no formation of humoral antibodies. On first exposure, T-cells become activated either by direct interaction with the specific antigen or by stimulation by an APC. The activated T-cells undergo proliferative expansion and maturation into sensitized T-cell and memory cells.

On subsequent exposure, the memory T-cells interact with the antigen and elicit an inflammatory response by the release of cytokines that exert an effect on the surrounding tissue. This response is amplified by the recruitment and activation of other effector cells to the target tissue. Because the reaction requires the clonal proliferation of the memory cells and subsequent release of cytokines, it is also called delayed hypersensitivity. An example of this type of reaction is contact dermatitis caused by plants from the genus *Rhus* (e.g., poison ivy, oak).

3. Nonspecific Immunity

Nonspecific (pharmacologic) immunity refers to initiation of inflammatory reactions by the nonspecific activation of cellular and humoral effector mechanisms without the formation of specific antibodies or antigen-specific sensitization of T-cells (CMI). A variety of compounds, including many biogenic substances, are capable of directly stimulating many types of cells (polyclonal cell activators). This type of reaction is discussed in Chapter 3 of this manual in describing the response to Gram-negative bacterial (GNB) endotoxin.

The inflammatory reactions are often identical to those observed from humoral or cell-mediated reactions; however, nonspecific immune reactions do not share the characteristics of memory and specificity.

B. Immune Hypersensitivity Reactions

Although the immune system normally has a protective role under some circumstances, its functioning can result in responses that damage the host. Repeated exposure to an antigen, for example, can induce an excessive immune response called hypersensitivity, which includes allergic asthma and rhinitis, hypersensitivity pneumonitis, and contact dermatitis. Other adverse immune responses include autoimmune reactions and immunosuppression.

The following comments will focus on hypersensitivity reactions since this is the type of adverse immune reaction associated most frequently with exposure to biogenic substances in the workplace. The different types of hypersensitivity reactions have been classified into four major categories. They are: Type I — immediate hypersensitivity reactions; Type II — cytotoxic reactions; Type III — immune complex reactions; and Type IV — cellular immunity.[1]

Type I (immediate hypersensitivity) reactions develop in sensitized individuals immediately after a second contact with the original sensitizing antigen. At primary sensitization, an antigen-specific IgE antibody is produced that can bind to surface receptors on basophils and mast cells.

If on subsequent exposure the specific antigen interacts with two adjacent IgE molecules on the cell surface, the cell integrity is altered — resulting in the release of rapidly acting mediators such as histamine. This response generally occurs rapidly on exposure to the offending antigen; however, other response patterns might be observed, including a late (delayed 4–8 hr) or dual (immediate and late) pattern. The delayed pattern is not to be confused with CMI. Depending on the target organ, the host may respond with bronchospasm, rhinitis, or urticaria.

Occupational asthma is defined as variable airflow limitation (a reversible bronchospasm) caused by a specific agent in the workplace. This definition is controversial because it includes substances that cause airflow limitation but are not sensitizers (see "Nonspecific Immunity" above).

Immunologically based occupational asthma is generally associated with a Type I response mediated by the antibody (IgE). Differentiation between immunologic and nonimmunologic or nonspecific airflow limitation is difficult and requires the demonstration of specific IgE antibody by an appropriate serological procedure.

Occupational asthma is caused by a variety of airborne agents, including low molecular weight chemicals and plant and animal products. Most of these materials are encountered in the industrial workplace, but the agents can also be found in other work environments such as research laboratories and contaminated indoor air. The overall prevalence of occupational asthma is unknown, but estimates range between 5%–15% of all cases of asthma.[2]

In **Type II** reactions, the antigen is associated with the surface of a cell: either as a surface protein or a low molecular weight substance (hapten) such as trimellitic anhydride that binds to a cell surface protein. On re-exposure, circulating IgG or IgM antibodies bind to the cell surface antigen, which initiates a series of events that results in the destruction of the cell. Hemolytic anemia and Goodpasture's disease have been associated with this type of response. Type II reactions have rarely been associated with exposure to biogenic substances.

Type III reactions occur when a soluble antigen binds with soluble IgG or IgM antibodies. This binding activates complement (a complex of enzymatic proteins in normal serum) which results in the formation of local immune complexes (e.g., Arthus reaction) or circulating immune complexes (e.g., serum sickness).

Some investigators have suggested that hypersensitivity pneumonitis (HP) — as characterized by pigeon breeders disease — is a Type III reaction. On primary exposure by inhalation to antigens in pigeon feces, specific IgG and IgM antibodies develop in the susceptible host. On subsequent exposure, localized immune complexes (Ag-Ab complexes) form in the lung. These complexes, which can activate complement, may result in the inflammatory reactions characteristic of hypersensitivity pneumonitis.

Type IV (delayed hypersensitivity) reactions, were described previously in the section on CMI. Some investigators have suggested that hypersensitivity pneumonitis is caused by a Type IV reaction; still others suggest there are two phases to HP: an initial nonspecific inflammation followed by an immune mediated reaction. In occupational environments, Type IV reactions have been associated most frequently with contact dermatitis (e.g., nickel).

Although it is convenient to place the immune reactions into discrete categories,[1] it should be acknowledged that exposure to specific biogenic substances can result in a combination of reactions. For a more detailed review of the field of immunology, a recently published textbook on immunology should be consulted. Table XV contains a partial listing of biological agents shown to cause occupational immunologic responses.

Table XV. Antigens of Biogenic Origin

Occupational Asthma: Allergic Mechanism, High Molecular Weight Compounds

Agents		Occupations
Animal products, insects, others		
Laboratory animals:	Rats, mice, rabbits, guinea pigs	Laboratory workers, veterinarians, animal handlers
Birds:	Pigeon, budgerigar	Pigeon breeders, poultry workers, bird fanciers
	Chicken	
Insects:	Grain mite	Grain workers
	Locust	Research laboratory
	River fly	Power plant along rivers
	Screw worm fly	Flight crews
	Cockroach	Laboratory workers
	Cricket	Field contact
	Bee moth	Fish bait breeders
	Moth and Butterfly	Entomologists
Plants		
Grain Dust		Grain handlers
Wheat/rye flour		Bakers, millers
Buckwheat		Bakers
Coffee beans		Food processors
Castor bean		Oil industry
Tea		Teaworker
Tobacco leaf		Tobacco manufacturing
Hops (*Humulus lupulus*)		Brewery chemist
Wood dust		
Western red cedar (*Thuja plicata*)		Carpenter, construction, cabinet maker, sawmill worker
California redwood		
Cedar of Lebanon		
Cocobolla		
Iroko		
Oak		
Mahogany		
Abiruana		
African maple		
Tanganyika aningre		
Central American walnut		
Kejaat		
African zebra wood		

Agents	Occupations
Microorganisms and Products	
B. subtilis	Detergent industry
Fungal amylase	Manufacturing, bakers
Gum Tragacanth	Gum manufacturing
Others	
Crab	Crab processing
Prawns	Prawn processing
Hoya	Oyster farm
Larva of silkworm	Sericulture

C. Measurement of Aeroallergens

Relatively few studies have evaluated the levels of airborne antigens in environments with biogenic antigens. Sample collection methods for aeroallergens do not differ from the methods used for gravimetric dust. The major limitation has been the lack of sensitive and reliable methods to identify specific antigens. Historically, three methods were used to estimate the concentrations of aeroallergens: 1) microscopic counting of pollen and mold spores; 2) evaluation of viable bioaerosols; and 3) chemical evaluations of specific antigens (such as isocyanates) or antigenic surrogates such as protein content.[3]

With the development of sensitive immunoassay techniques, low concentrations of specific antigens can be measured by extracting gravimetric dust samples. Variables that influence the recovery and detection of aeroallergens include volume of air sampled; filter extraction efficiency; and the sensitivity of the assay. Accurate quantitation requires the reference antigen to have the same specificity as the target antigen, and that the assay is not affected by substances that might be present in environments with organic dust.

At publication of this manual, there were no approved or standardized protocols for the evaluation of exposure to airborne antigens. Until such protocols are proposed, evaluated, and standardized, it is recommended that a person trained in medicine and immunology be consulted to develop a strategy for evaluating exposure to airborne antigens.

The majority of studies evaluating specific aeroallergens have focused either on domestic indoor environments or animal laboratory containment facilities. Environmental variables shown to influence the concentration of aeroallergens include particle size; humidity; density of animals; and socioeconomic factors.[3]

D. Exposure to Occupational Allergens

In developing practices and procedures directed to the control of hazards in the workplace, emphasis usually is placed on those elements that present an immediate or serious hazard to personnel or to the environment. Often, however, little attention is given to hazards that might result in illnesses of low incidence or of nondisabling consequence. Allergies fall into each of these broad categories, although to the person affected an allergy can cause significant health problems and result in loss of income. Many environments exists in which exposure to occupational allergens can occur. These include, but are not limited to, workers in the food industry, pharmaceutical industry, and the agriculture and textile industries.

As an approach to alerting personnel to this potential hazard and in the interest of providing some insight into the problems of allergies in employees, allergies to animal dander is discussed below as an example of an environment with occupational exposure to allergens. Exposure to animal dander occurs primarily in the research laboratory setting. The major difference between industry and the research laboratory is the amount of allergen to which the worker is exposed.

1. Animal Dander Allergies

Laboratory animal dander allergies (LADA) are generally defined as Type I reactions mediated by an IgE antibody, caused by dermal or inhalation exposure to animal fur, saliva, urine, or other body products. Outcomes associated with inhalation exposure include rhinitis, conjunctivitis, and wheezing and cough (asthma). Dermal symptoms include urticaria and angioedema. Lutsky and Neuman reported that 70% of persons with LADA responded with symptoms within 5 min of exposure to allergens and that 93% responded within 10 min.[4] Various symptoms were reported, including rhinitis/conjunctivitis (100%), asthma (71%), cough (58%), and palatal itch (38%). Lincoln et al. reported similar findings: rhinitis/conjunctivitis (81%), asthma (48%), mild wheezing (30%), angioedema (7%), and various skin reactions such as hives and eczema (56%).[5] They also reported that some of the persons in the study demonstrated contact sensitivity (hives) to rodent urine or blood.

Although researchers have known about LADAs for many years, little was known about their frequency until the mid-70s. Lutsky and Neuman[4] found that of 1293 workers exposed to laboratory animals, 191 (14.7%) became hypersensitive to dander. The animal facilities were located in medical schools, research institutes, universities, pharmaceutical manufacturers, veterinary colleges, commercial animal producer facilities, and hospitals. One study found that 27 of 238 persons (11.3%) having extensive contact with animals at Oak Ridge National Laboratory were hypersensitive to animal dander.[5] The rates reported in the two studies are within the 10%–20% range of allergic phenomena reported for the general population of the United States.[6] More recent publications, however, tend to indicate higher incidence rates up to 30% for LADA.[7]

In the study by Lincoln et al., it is of interest to note that allergies were observed more frequently in staff scientists and laboratory technicians than in animal caretakers or custodians (see Table XVI).[5] Table XVII shows that the incidence of allergy (by history and/or a positive skin test) was higher in thosewith a college education or graduate degrees than in those with a high school education or less. Several explanations have been offered to account for this trend (i.e., the more highly educated group is less tolerant of allergy symptoms and gives more detailed histories; that technical level personnel select themselves out of allergy-producing occupations; or that workers with higher education have taken years to develop a career and are reluctant to leave).[4,8] Lincoln et al. suggest that all beginning graduate students in disciplines involving animal contact be carefully evaluated by obtaining a complete medical history and thorough skin testing.[5] Thus, sensitized persons entering a discipline involving extensive animal contact would have an opportunity to re-evaluate their professional goals.

Table XVI. Distribution of LADA[A] Among 238 Employees According to Job Title[B]

Job Title	No.
Research scientist	15
Technicians	10
Animal attendants/custodians	2
Administrative staff	0
Clerical staff	0

[A] LADA = laboratory animal dander allergies.

[B] Source: **Lincoln, T.A., N.E. Bolton, and A.S. Garrett:** Occupational Allergy to Animal Dander and Sera. *J. Occup. Med. 16*:465-469 (1974).

Table XVII. History and Skin Test Results According to Education[A]

History	Skin Test	College or Graduate	High School or Less
+	+	24.7%	11.8%
+	−	10.4%	11.0%
−	+	15.3%	18.6%
−	−	49.4%	58.4%

+ = reported allergy in a medical history

− = allergy not reported in the history

[A] Source: **Lincoln, T.A., N.E. Bolton, and A.S. Garrett:** Occupational Allergy to Animal Dander and Sera. *J. Occup. Med. 16*:465-469 (1974).

The development of LADA symptoms varies from less than one year to many years after initial contact. According to Lutsky and Neuman, symptoms develop in one year or less for 38% of those affected, in two years for 10%, in three years for 24%, and in four or more years for 28%.[4] The data indicate that a longer period of time is required for LADA to develop in those without a history of allergy or a positive skin test to a variety of allergens. Persons with an atopic predisposition as determined by history or skin test are at an increased risk of developing LADA; however, the degree of risk is undefined. Lincoln et al. found that 50% of the sensitized employees had relatives with allergy and 52% had seasonal allergic rhinitis that was exacerbated by exposure to animals.[5] When these employees were skin-tested (prick test), 8% were found to be sensitive to pollens, 63% to house dust, and 89% to various animal danders. Other studies have shown similar responses.[9-16]

Persons with LADA are often hypersensitive to more than one species of animal. One study reported that 55% of the subjects were allergic to two or more animals;[4] another study reported a similar observation in 45% of evaluated subjects.[12] The cat (16%) was the animal most frequently associated with animal allergies, followed by the rabbit (14.6%), guinea pigs (12.8%), and rats (11.6%). Most LADA are associated with small mammals such as rats, mice, guinea pigs, and rabbits.[9]

Sensitivity might be highly specific for certain strains of animals. Sorrel and Gottesman[17] reported severe rhinitis in an individual after a few months exposure to C-57 and C-58 Swiss mice, although the individual had worked with other species of mice for many years. There seemed to be no history of allergy, but the individual had a positive reaction to C-57 and C-58 dander in a scratch test. The reaction to a commercial mouse skin test antigen was weak. Voorhorst[18] described two animal handlers who developed severe allergic symptoms when a group of agoutic rodents were introduced into the animal colony, although both technicians had worked with a variety of rodents for many years without symptoms of allergy.

Exposure of animal urine via direct contact or inhalation of contaminated dusts (dander, hair, bedding, etc.) is prevalent in various aspects of animal handling. Lincoln et al. concluded that aerosolized dander and urine were more important sources of allergen than food or bedding because the latter are aerosolized in limited amounts as rather large particles that settle rapidly.[5] Their data suggest that soluble protein material on dander is as important as or more so than the dander itself. More recent studies suggest proteins from saliva and urine represent the greatest risk for LADA.[19-21] Urine proteins from rats and mice are more potent because of their nonvolatile, high molecular weight characteristics.[21]

Direct contact with animals is not necessary for the development of LADA. Sensitivity to rat dander was reported in a 5-year-old whose only contact was through his mother, a research assistant having daily contact with rodents.[18] This case emphasizes the need for personal hygiene, personal protective equipment (PPE), and appropriate facilities in the workplace to prevent secondary exposures in addition to reducing the severity of symptoms in the primary contact. Perhaps a shower at the end of the workday would benefit both the patient and atopic relatives.

Taken together, the results of these studies permit construction of a LADA profile. The patient is an employee of either sex, a scientific or technical worker, 28 to 32 years old, has a family history of atopy, develops hypersensitivity within three years of animal contact, has an immediate type response (less than 10 min), displays three or more clinical symptoms (most frequently rhinitis, asthma, and cough) and is sensitive to one or two animal species.

The effect of LADA on employment can be serious. Although 75% of atopic individuals in the study by Lutsky and Neuman[4] could continue their work using masks and antihistamines, 28% either changed jobs or avoided specific animals. Of the latter 28%, half voluntarily resigned their jobs. Lincoln et al. found that 37% of atopic employees either avoided exposure altogether or wore a respirator.[5] Some technicians were reassigned; others adjusted their work schedules to allow only brief exposures to animals.

Three major approaches have been recommended to reduce exposure or minimize the effects of exposure:[5]
  a. Pre-employment evaluation to identify workers at increased risk.
  b. Personal protective measures: This includes the use of gown or lab coat, vinyl or rubber gloves, approved disposable dust respirators and shoe covers. Care should be taken to assure proper fit of respirators and gloves. If garments are used in handling animals, they should be either disposable and discarded on exiting the animal room. If reusable garments are used, appropriate handling guidelines must be implemented. The efficacy of such personal protective measures is difficult to determine, although subjective observations suggest they help reduce the frequency and severity of symptoms in affected individuals.

c. Methods to reduce antigen release: The use of filter-top cages or other updated designs (e.g., HEPA-filtered cages, filtered laminar flow cage racks, use of wire floors in rodent cages to eliminate wood chip bedding and reduce dust emissions, and cage systems with automatic flushing systems); biological safety cabinets for handling animals or cage-emptying; a well-designed ventilation system (both local exhaust and dilution ventilation); independent room ventilation with special ceiling to floor airflow with positive air pressure in animal rooms; and use of dust-free bedding.

2. Industrial Enzymes

Enzymes are proteins that serve as catalysts in biochemical reactions. They are naturally occurring products (e.g., derived from a variety of animal, plant, and microbial sources) that can be produced in commercial quantities either through extraction from natural sources by chemical or mechanical methods, or by fermentation processes. Their structure determines both functionality and human antigenic potential.

Occupationally, the most studied type of enzymes have been bacterial proteases that break down various protein substrates into less complex polypeptide units. These enzymes have been widely used in laundry detergents. The information in this chapter is provided as a general overview of current health and safety issues related to the industrial production and use of these enzymes. This chapter should be used only as a guide to this topic. The reader is referred to the references at the end of this chapter for more detailed information. The practices described should be generally applicable to operations involving nonproteolytic enzymes.

It is important to remember that commercially available enzymes are derived from nontoxicogenic, nonpathogenic microorganisms and the producing strains are not carried over into the finished product in a viable state.

3. Health Effects

Proteolytic enzymes cause eye irritation and are capable of causing nonallergic skin irritation (on repeated or prolong contact with unprotected skin). Their greatest potential health risk, however, is immunologic sensitization. Enzymes, like other naturally occurring proteins, are capable of initiating antibody production (sero-conversion) and Type I IgE mediated allergic responses in exposed individuals.

Sero-conversion due to enzyme exposure is known to occur only as a result of inhalation. There is no evidence to indicate that skin contact will result in systemic IgE mediated sero-conversion and subsequent allergic response.

Sero-conversion does not necessarily result in the appearance of clinical symptoms. Within any population, a portion of those who develop antibodies will develop clinical symptoms with additional exposure to enzymes. The clinical symptoms are the same as those associated with classical hay fever or ragweed pollen allergies. The clinical response, and the propensity to initially develop antibodies, has been shown to be somewhat conditional on still undefined individual predisposition factors in addition to exposure dose.

There is no evidence that commercially available enzyme preparations have mutagenic, teratogenic, or carcinogenic potential by any route of exposure or level of dose.

4. Exposure Limits

ACGIH has established a ceiling threshold limit value (TLV) of 0.00006 mg/m^3 (60 ng/m^3) for proteolytic enzymes (subtilisins) derived from *B. subtilis* or closely related species.[22] This exposure limit is based on 100% pure crystalline enzyme. The ceiling limit is based on high volume sampling for 60 min because of the analytical limitations at the time the TLV was established.

5. Enzyme Exposure Control

The exposure routes of concern associated with industrial enzyme products are, in order of importance, inhalation, and skin/eye contact; therefore, any control strategy designed to reduce employee exposure must concern itself with the reduction or elimination of aerosol generation and opportunities for direct eye, skin, or mucous membrane contact.

Careful attention to the design, location, and maintenance of exhaust ventilation in conjunction with carefully developed work practices have proved effective in the reduction of occupational exposures.

6.   Personal Protective Equipment and Hygiene Practices

Although good work practices and engineering controls will reduce the need for personal protective equipment during routine operations, there are activities that require PPE, including respiratory protection, to control potential employee exposure. It is not uncommon for PPE to be used combined with engineering controls and workplace practices during equipment cleaning, scheduled maintenance activities, enzyme-product spill cleanup, and emergency response activities.

7.   Exposure Monitoring

There are several reports of sampling and analytical methods for evaluating airborne levels of enzymes in the work environment.[23-28] All of these analytical methods are for subtilisins or papain. The ACGIH TLV for subtilisins and its interpretation is based on area sampling using a high flow pump (400–600 L/min) and analysis by enzyme activity assays.

Enzymes have unique biological and chemical properties that present challenges when developing air monitoring and assay methods. Enzymes are large biological molecules that will become inactive if not handled properly. Stability is of particular concern during air monitoring and storage. Enzymes are classified by their function, and each class is composed of multiple entities with unique specific activities and antigenic properties. Subtilisins, for example, are a group of serine proteases that degrade proteins.

For many years proteases have been measured with an activity assay using a natural substrate, N,N,-dimethyl casein. This method has been described by Dunn and Brotherton[23] and Bruce et al.[28] Drawbacks to this method include low sensitivity and nonspecificity. A high volume sample must be taken to obtain a sufficient sample for analysis; thus, personal sampling cannot be used to assess exposure levels. The assay cannot distinguish between different subtilisins, so it can only be used when one subtilisin is present. It is critical that the particular reference subtilisin be used in the analysis.

Increased sensitivity via a fluoresamine method was described by Chein in 1978.[24] Rothgeb also reported increased sensitivity with a synthetic substrate, p-nitroanilide.[27] The Rothgeb method is sensitive enough for personal sampling. These two methods did not improve specificity and cannot be used when more than one subtilisin is present.

In 1981, Wells et al. described an immunoassay for papain measurement in the industrial setting.[25] This was followed in 1986 by a similar method for a subtilisin.[26] These methods require isotopes and a radiobiology lab to perform the assay. At the 1990 American Industrial Hygiene Conference (AIHC) in Orlando, Fla., a paper was presented on an Enzyme-Linked ImmunoSorbent Assay (ELISA) for quantitating a protein. These methods are based on antigen-antibody reactions, which greatly improve the sensitivity and specificity of previous assays. The principal drawbacks are the relative difficulty in obtaining a key reagent, purified anti-sera from an immunized animal host, and specialized analytical equipment is required. A specific anti-sera must be obtained for each enzyme to be analyzed.

8.   Medical Surveillance Programs

The purpose of medical monitoring is to protect employee health through the early identification of occupational health problems. It is recommended that such a program be implemented whenever enzymes are handled.

A medical surveillance program for facilities that handle enzymes should include:

a. Preplacement evaluations to establish baseline health status and to identify individuals who might be more prone to developing adverse health effects when working with enzymes;
b. Periodic evaluations to identify individuals who have experienced sero-conversions and/or adverse health effects from exposure to enzymes.

The information provided from a medical surveillance program can be used to evaluate the effectiveness of engineering controls, PPE, and employee training.

There are two medical tests that can be conducted to determine whether an individual has developed antibodies to a specific enzyme. Antibodies can be detected either through a laboratory blood test (such as a RAST)[29,30] or by a simple skin prick test commonly used by allergists.[31,32] Blood and skin tests only provide presumptive evidence that a person has sero-converted and has developed antibodies to the specific enzyme tested, and not that this person will exhibit clinical allergy symptoms.

References

1. **Coombs, R.A., and P.G.H. Gell:** Classification of Allergic Reactions Responsible for Clinical Hypersensitivity and Disease. In *Clinical Aspects of Immunology* (edited by P.G.H. Gell, R.A. Coombs, and P.J. Lachmann). Blackwell Scientific Publications, 1975. pp. 761-781.

2. **Chang-Yeung, M., and S. Lam:** Occupational Asthma. *Am. Rev. Respir. Dis. 133:*686-703 (1986).

3. **Newman-Taylor, A., and R.D. Tee:** Environmental and Occupational Asthma — Exposure Assessment. *Chest 98(5):*209S-211S (1990).

4. **Lutsky, I.I., and I. Neuman:** Laboratory Animal Dander Allergy (I. An Occupational Disease). *Ann. Allergy 35:*201-205 (1975).

5. **Lincoln, T.A., N.E. Bolton, and A.S. Garrett:** Occupational Allergy to Animal Dander and Sera. *J. Occup. Med. 16:*465-469 (1974).

6. **Tennenbaum, J.I.:** Immunology and Allergy. In *Genetic Disorders of Man* (edited by R.M. Goodman). Boston: Little, Brown and Co., 1970.

7. **Slovak, A.J.M., and R.N. Hill:** Laboratory Animal Allergy: A Clinical Survey of an Exposed Population. *Brit. J. Ind. Med. 38:*38-41 (1981).

8. **Gross, N.J.:** Allergy to Laboratory Animals: Epidemiologic, Clinical and Physiologic Aspects and a Trial of Cromolyn in its Management. *J. Allergy Clin. Immunol. 66:*158-165 (1980).

9. **Agrup, G., L. Belin, L. Sjostedt, and S. Skerfving:** Allergy to Laboratory Animals in Laboratory Technicians and Animal Keepers. *Brit. J. Ind. Med. 43:*192-198 (1986).

10. **Barbee, R.A., M.D. Lebowitz, H.C. Thompson, and B. Burrows:** Immediate Skin-Test Reactivity in a General Population Sample. *Ann. Intern. Med. 84:*129 (1976).

11. **Bartholeme, K., W. Kissler, H. Boer, E. Koiiett-Schulte, and U. Wahr:** Where Does Cat Allergen Come From? *J. Allergy Clin. Immunol. 76:*503-506 (1985).

12. **Bland, S.M., M.S. Levine, P.D. Wilson, N.L. Fox, and J.C. Rivera:** Occupational Allergy to Laboratory Animals: An Epidemiologic Study. *J. Occup. Med. 28:*1151-1157 (1986).

13. **Cockcroft, A., J. Edwards, P. McCarthy, and N. Andersson:** Allergy in Laboratory Animal Workers. *Lancet 1:*827-830 (1981).

14. **Davies, G.E., and L.A. McArdle:** Allergy to Laboratory Animals: A Survey by Questionnaire. *Arch. Allergy Appl. Immunol. 64:*302 (1981).

15. **Davies, G.E., A.V. Thompson, Z. Niewola, G.E. Burrows, E.L. Teaschle, D.J. Bird, and D.A. Phillips:** Allergy to Laboratory Animals: A Retrospective and a Prospective Study. *Brit. J. Ind. Med. 40:*442-449 (1983).

16. **Newman-Taylor, A.J., J.R. Myers, J.L. Longbottom, D. Spackman, and A.J.M. Slovak:** Immunological Differences Between Asthma and Other Allergic Reactions in Laboratory Workers. *Thorax 36:*229 (1981). [Abstract.]

17. **Sorrell, A.H., and J. Gottesman:** Mouse Allergy — A Case Report. *Ann. Allergy 15:*662-663 (1957).

18. **Voorhorst, R.:** The Dander-Allergens as a Cause of Vasomotor Rhinitis. *Int. Rhinol. 3:*65 (1965).

19. **Levy, D.A., M. Ohi, and C.Y. Pascual:** Allergenic Activity of Rat Saliva. *Monogr. Allergy 18:*144 (1983).

20. **Newman-Taylor, A.J., J.R. Myers, J.L. Longbottom, and J. Pepys:** Respiratory Allergy to Urine Proteins of Rats and Mice. *Lancet 2:*847-849 (1977).

21. **Walls, A.F., and J.L. Longbottom:** Comparison of Rat Fur, Urine, Saliva and Other Rat Allergen Extracts by Skin Testing, RAST, and RAST Inhibition. *J. Allergy Clin. Immunol. 75:*242 (1985).

22. **American Conference of Governmental Industrial Hygienists:** *1993-1994 Threshold Limit Values for Chemical Substances and Physical Agents and Biological Exposure Indices.* Cincinnati, Ohio: American Conference of Governmental Industrial Hygienists, 1993. p. 32.

23. **Dunn, E., and R. Brotherton:** The Use of N,N,-dimethylcasein in the Determination of Proteolytic Enzymes in Washing Products and Airborne Dust Samples. *Analyst 96:*159-163 (1971).

24. **Chien, P.T.:** The Development of a Fluorometric Method for the Assay of Subtilisins. *Am. Ind. Hyg. Assoc. J. 39(10):*808-816 (1978).

25. **Wells, I.D., R.E. Allan, H.S. Hovey, and B.D. Culner:** Detection of Airborne Industrial Papain by a Radioimmunoassay. *Am. Ind. Hyg. Assoc. J. 42(4):*321-322 (1981).

26. **Agarwal, M.K., J.W. Ingram, S. Dunnette, and G.J. Gleich:** Immunochemical Quantitation of an Airborne Proteolytic Enzyme, Esperase®, in a Consumer Products Factory. *Am. Ind. Hyg. Assoc. J. 47(2):*138-143 (1986).

27. **Rothgeb, T.M., B.D. Goodlander, P.H. Garrison, and L.A. Smith:** The Raw Material, Finished Products and Dust Pad Analysis of Detergent Proteases Using a Small Synthetic Substrate. *JAOCS 65:*806-810 (1988).

28. **Bruce, C.F., E. Dunn, R. Brotherton, D.R. Davies, F. Hall, and S.C.M. Potts:** Methods of Measuring Biologically Active Enzyme Dust in the Environmental Air of Detergent Factories. *Ann. Occup. Hyg. 21:*1-20 (1978).

29. **Doll, N.J., B.E. Bozelka, and J.E. Salvaggio:** Immunology and Immunodiagnostic Tests. In *Environmental and Occupational Medicine.* Boston: Little, Brown and Co., 1983. pp. 52-53.

30. **Newman, L., E. Storey, and K. Kreiss:** Immunologic Evaluation. In *Occupational Medicine State of the Art Reviews: Occupational Pulmonary Disease.* Philadelphia: Hanley and Belfus, Inc., 1987. pp. 345-372.

31. **Belin, L.G.A., and P.S. Norman:** Diagnostic Tests in the Skin and Serum of Workers Sensitized to Bacillus Subtilis Enzymes. *Clinical Allergy 7:*55-68 (1977).

32. **Pepys, J.:** Skin Testing. *Brit. J. Hosp. Med. 32(3):*120-124 (1984).

5. Control Methods

A. Introduction

The term "biosafety" describes a complete program of administrative controls, medical surveillance, vaccination (when appropriate), and containment strategies for reducing the risk of disease in laboratory workers and other persons with potential exposure to infectious agents or other biologically derived molecules. Containment strategies include methods to protect the worker from exposure to biological agents and to prevent the release of such agents into the outside environment. The three elements of containment include laboratory practice and technique, safety equipment, and facility design. As a means of specifying these elements in biomedical and research lab settings, a biosafety level (BSL) rating has been formulated by the Centers for Disease Control and Prevention.* BSLs have also been used in biotechnology and animal care facilities and can be applied theoretically in any occupational setting.

B. Biosafety Levels

There are four biosafety levels for infectious agents. These biosafety levels, which consist of combinations of laboratory practices and techniques, safety equipment, and laboratory facilities appropriate for the hazards posed by handling infectious agents, are described in greater detail in Appendix II.

Biosafety Level 1 (BSL1) practices, safety equipment, and facilities are appropriate for undergraduate and secondary educational training and teaching laboratories, and for other facilities in which work is done with defined and characterized strains of viable microorganisms not known to cause disease in healthy adult humans. *Bacillus subtilis*, *Naegleria gruberi*, and infectious canine hepatitis virus are examples of microorganisms meeting these criteria. Many agents not ordinarily associated with disease processes in humans, however, are opportunistic pathogens and may cause infection in the young, the aged, and in immunodeficient or immunosuppressed individuals. Vaccine strains that have undergone multiple *in vivo* passages should not be considered avirulent simply because they are vaccine strains.

Biosafety Level 2 (BSL2) practices, safety equipment, and facilities are applicable to clinical, diagnostic, teaching, and other facilities in which work is done with the broad spectrum of indigenous moderate-risk agents present in the community and associated with human disease of varying severity. With good microbiological techniques, these agents can be used safely in activities conducted on the open bench, provided the potential for producing aerosols is low. Hepatitis B virus, the *Salmonella* spp., and *Toxoplasma* spp. are representative of microorganisms assigned to this containment level. Primary hazards to personnel working with these agents may include accidental autoinoculation, ingestion, and skin or mucous membrane exposure to infectious materials. Procedures with high aerosol potential must be conducted in primary containment equipment or devices.

Biosafety Level 3 (BSL3) practices, safety equipment, and facilities are applicable to clinical, diagnostic, teaching, research, or production facilities in which work is done with indigenous or exotic agents where the potential for infection by aerosols is real and the disease might have serious or lethal consequences. Autoinoculation and ingestion represent the primary hazards to personnel working with these agents. Examples of such agents for which Biosafety Level 3 safeguards generally are recommended include *Mycobacterium tuberculosis*, St. Louis encephalitis virus, and *Coxiella burnetii*.

---

* The abbreviations BSL and BL for biosafety level are used interchangeably by various organizations and government agencies. For consistency, BSL is being used in this manual.

Biosafety Level 4 (BSL4) practices, safety equipment, and facilities are applicable to work with dangerous and exotic agents that pose a high individual risk of life-threatening disease. All manipulations of potentially infectious diagnostic materials, isolates, and naturally or experimentally infected animals pose a high risk of exposure and infection to laboratory personnel. Lassa fever virus is representative of the agents assigned to Level 4.

Biosafety levels are also described for activities involving experimental animals. These four combinations of practices, safety equipment, and facilities are designated animal biosafety levels (ABSL) 1, 2, 3, and 4 and provide increasing levels of protection to personnel and the environment. These are described in detail in Appendix III, which also includes a listing of zoonotic diseases and a list of specific organisms isolated from urine and feces of infected animals.

Containment for large-scale recombinant DNA experiments or production, greater than 10 L, is described in the National Institutes of Health (NIH) *Guidelines for Research Involving Recombinant DNA Molecules*[1] and in the Organisation for Economic Co-operation and Development's *Safety Considerations for Biotechnology.*[2] NIH describes four levels of large scale containment: Good Large Scale Practices (GLSP), Biosafety Level 1 Large Scale (BSL1–LS), Biosafety Level 2 Large Scale (BSL2–LS), and Biosafety Level 3 Large Scale (BSL3–LS). These large scale guidelines could also be applied to experiments and production of nonrecombinant organisms. The criteria for large scale containment are described in Appendix IV.

C. Work Practices and Techniques

The most important element of containment is strict adherence to standard microbiological practices and techniques.

1. Administrative Controls

Program Administrator: Qualified individuals must do the following in management of an effective biosafety program:

- Supervise the safety performance of the employees to ensure that the required safety practices and techniques are used;
- Develop emergency plans for spills and personnel contamination;
- Instruct and train employees in the practices and techniques required to ensure safety;
- Ensure the integrity of the physical and biological containment;
- Inform employees of the medical surveillance program;
- Correct work errors and conditions that might result in exposure or release;
- Select appropriate microbiological practices and techniques;
- Ensure periodic workplace evaluations; and
- Interact with the workplace biosafety committee (see below).

These responsibilities may be assigned jointly to the direct supervisor, laboratory director, biosafety officer, or other health and safety professionals.

Each workplace is unique and requires biosafety programs tailored to meet specific needs. The program administrator is responsible for selecting additional safety practices, which must be consistent with the hazards associated with the agent or procedure. As a general policy, clinical, field, and environmental specimens should be handled at the level recommended for the most pathogenic agent that the clinical diagnosis or other evidence suggests is likely to be present. For example, sputa submitted to the laboratory should be handled from the outset as potentially infectious for tuberculosis. Personnel working with specimens or tissues submitted for rabies examination should be immunized and take appropriate precautions to prevent parenteral or aerosol exposures. Personnel working with specimens or tissues of domestic and wild animals shouldbe aware of known or potential zoonotic infections, should be immunized if vaccines are available, and should observe other common sense precautionary measures. Personnel working with human neural tissue should take precautions against Creutzfeldt-Jakob agent.

Employee's Role: The success or failure of any biohazards control program ultimately rests with the employee. Each employee is responsible for complying with all safety rules, regulations, and procedures required for the task assigned. He or she also is responsible for reporting all facts to the immediate supervisor regarding accidents resulting in personal injury, illness, and/or property damage and any actions or conditions that could result in such incidents.

Biosafety Committee: Workplaces that handle biohazardous agents should have a standing biosafety committee. Members of this committee should have broad backgrounds in microbiology, medicine (human and veterinary), industrial hygiene, engineering, and occupational safety. Biosafety committees are responsible for defining the potential risk of planned work associated with the use of biohazardous agents.

Biosafety Manuals and Training: Each organization that works with biohazardous agents should develop a biosafety operations manual specific for that facility which identifies the hazards that will or might be encountered. The manual should specify practices and procedures designed to minimize or eliminate risks. Personnel should be advised of special hazards and should be required to read and follow the required practices and procedures. Information and training programs should be developed and initially provided for all employees. New employees should receive training prior to beginning work, and refresher courses should be available to all employees at risk of exposure on an annual basis, if not more frequently.

Use of a Universal Biohazard Warning Sign: Establishment of policies and procedures for identification and control of biological hazards is another form of administrative control. Proper identification of

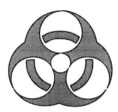

hazardous biological agents is necessary to alert support personnel who may enter the area to take precautionary measures and to restrict traffic to hazardous areas. It is the primary responsibility of the supervisor/laboratory director to identify biohazards properly. To ensure proper identification of biological hazards, a standardized, easily recognized sign is essential. The warning sign must be placed so that it can be seen easily and displayed *only* for the purpose of indicating the presence of actual or potential biological hazards. The biohazard warning symbol shown in Figure 2 must appear on the door sign.

Figure 2. Universal biohazard symbol.

2.   Medical Surveillance

Application of traditional industrial hygiene sampling and exposure assessment techniques for hazard evaluation can be complicated by the following factors: 1) the consequences of exposure to many biohazards are hypothetical or unknown, and 2) the minimum dose for all but a few well-characterized biogenic agents is unknown; consequently, there are few occupational exposure limits. These uncertainties underscore the need for medical surveillance.[3]

Specific recommendations concerning the need for either preassignment or periodic medical examinations for workers engaged in biohazardous operations must be determined on a case-by-case basis. The recommendations will depend on the assessed hazards of the work and the individual needs of the worker.

Medical surveillance is focused on the early detection of illness or injury, therefore, is a form of secondary prevention.[3,4] Secondary prevention is the detection and termination of an illness before the worker normally would have sought medical care.[5] Medical surveillance has been used to monitor the effectiveness of exposure controls and the effectiveness of personal protective equipment. Other goals of medical surveillance include the identification of medical conditions that place the worker at increased risk of a work-related illness or injury,[6] documentation of the baseline and periodic health status of the workers, and data collection for future epidemiologic review. Table XVIII lists some other uses of medical surveillance, and Table XIX some limitations.

Table XVIII. Some Uses of Medical Surveillance *

• Provides evidence of exposure;

• Detects disease early;

• Assesses the efficacy of exposure control measures;

• Detects changes in the health of employees;

• Determines the suitability of an individual for a particular job due to physical attributes or sensitivities;

Table XVIII (continued). Some Uses of Medical Surveillance *

- Detects patterns of disease or subclinical parameters in the work force;
- Emphasizes the existence of job-related hazards to the workers;
- Establishes a medical and serological baseline;
- Maintains records;
- Ensures that at-risk workers are appropriately immunized;
- Identifies workers with greater likelihood of developing work-related illness (i.e., sensitivity screening)
- Determines suitability of employees for respirator use; and
- Meets regulatory requirements.

---

* Adapted from the following references:

Classification of Allergic Reactions Responsible for Clinical Hypersensitivity and Disease. In *Clinical Aspects of Immunology* (edited by P.G.H. Gell, R.A. Coombs, and P.J. Lachmann). Philadelphia: Blackwell Scientific Publications, 1975.

Chang-Yeung, M., and S. Lam: Occupational Asthma. *Am. Rev. Respir. Dis. 133:*686-703 (1986).

Agarwal, M.K., J.W. Ingram, S. Dunnette, and G.J. Gleich: Immunochemical Quantitation of an Airborne Proteolytic Enzyme, Esperase®, in a Consumer Products Factory. *Am. Ind. Hyg. Assoc. J. 47(2):*138-143 (1986).

Table XIX. Limitations of Medical Surveillance

- Groups are generally small in size;
- Exposures are variable;
- There can be a long latency period between exposure and disease;
- Effects of exposure frequently are uncertain;
- Most medical tests are nonspecific and nonselective;
- Tests may detect disease or injury only after serious and irreversible adverse health effects have developed;
- Some tests produce high false-positive and false-negative results; and
- It sometimes is difficult to distinguish occupational from nonoccupational causation.

The Medical Surveillance Process

Development of a medical surveillance program may include the following steps:
1) Identify the exposures and potentially exposed workers;
2) Characterize the potential health effects or hypersensitivities;
3) Select the medical surveillance instruments;
4) Perform medical surveillance;
5) Document data collection;
6) Analyze the data; and
7) Report the data and recommendations to workers and appropriate management.

1) Identify Exposures: The process of exposure identification involves characterizing the workplace, the work force, and the agents present and then using this information to develop homogeneous exposure groups.[7] All members of a homogeneous exposure group are presumed to have similar exposures and are at risk for similar health effects; therefore, they should receive identical medical surveillance. If developed carefully, these homogeneous exposure group designations may be useful in future epidemiological studies of the population.

2) Characterize Potential Health Effects: Characterize the potential health effects and signs of exposure to the agents to which each homogeneous exposure group is potentially exposed. Medical conditions that can reduce a worker's immunocompetence or detoxification systems should also be identified at this stage.

3-4) Select Medical Surveillance Instruments and Perform Medical Surveillance: The medical surveillance instruments must be specific for the health effects attributable to the agent(s) or to conditions believed to affect the worker's natural defenses.

Whether the instruments are administered monthly, annually, or at other intervals must match the progression of the expected health consequences of exposure. Most medical surveillance programs are composed of a baseline medical evaluation conducted at preplacement, periodic evaluations, a final evaluation upon leaving the work area, and special examinations in the event of spills, failures of containment equipment, or the development of work-related medical signs or symptoms.[4,6]

A CDC/NIOSH ad hoc working group convened by NIH to study medical surveillance for industrial applications of biotechnology[6] recommends that preplacement examinations be designed to:

- establish a worker's health status prior to employment;
- provide baseline data for possible epidemiological studies;
- identify conditions that make the worker more susceptible to work-related illness; and
- obtain data on risk factors.

These goals can be accomplished by obtaining a thorough medical and occupational history, and by conducting a physical examination and appropriate laboratory tests.[4,8] The elements of a physical examination and the selection of laboratory tests depends on the purpose of surveillance. Sullivan presented a thorough summary of available clinical laboratory tests that may be useful in medical surveillance of workers in biological research and biotechnology.[8] The elements of medical surveillance must also be practicable in the setting and be acceptableto the employees. All medical surveillance exams should be conducted in compliance with the Americans with Disabilities Act of 1992.

Periodic medical evaluations should include parameters that will provide useful information on the early effects of exposure and changes in natural defenses or the development of antibodies to specific antigens.[4] Comprehensive periodic physical examinations are generally of little value.[6]

For appropriate quality control of clinical laboratory tests, blank, spiked, or duplicate samples should be submitted periodically to the testing laboratory to document the quality of the analytical results. Equipment used in the physical examination (such as spirometers and audiometers) should be calibrated daily and serviced routinely.

The exit exam is given to workers who are leaving a particular homogeneous exposure group. The purpose of an exit exam is to allow a comparison of the health status of the worker at preplacement and at exit; therefore, it should resemble the preplacement exam.

Special medical examinations and follow-up procedures should be developed for workers:

- involved in spills, failures of engineering controls, or accidental exposures (such as needlesticks);[4]
- who have suffered from prolonged (> 48 hours) or unexplained illnesses;[6] or
- who develop health effects that are potentially work-related.

These examinations should look for early evidence of illness in those exposed or determine whether reported health effects are in any way related to agents in the workplace and whether similar health effects have been seen in co-workers. The results of these evaluations should be used to determine the need for further medical follow-up and whether modifications to existing engineering and work practice controls and other procedures are justified.

5) Document Data Collection: Data must be collected in a way that makes it easily retrievable and analyzable. The documentation from the exposure identification process and the development of the homogeneously exposed groups must be retained. All findings from physical examinations, questionnaire responses, and laboratory test results must be included as part of the worker's permanent medical record and should be formatted for meaningful evaluation. All equipment calibration, maintenance information, and quality control data must also be retained.

6) Analyze the Data: Collected data must be analyzed. Individual results should be compared with population norms, if available, and with previous and baseline results. Grouped data from individuals within a homogeneously exposed group can be periodically analyzed. In the long term, epidemiological analyses of accident or illness records, specific laboratory findings, and other morbidity and mortality information can be performed.

7) Give Report and Recommendations: All results of medical surveillance must be reported to the participating worker. Summaries of results by a homogeneously exposed group can be developed for the biosafety officer and facility management. Confidentiality of participating workers must be maintained.

Legal and Regulatory Requirements

OSHA has not specifically mandated biological monitoring or medical surveillance of workers potentially exposed to biological hazards (e.g., in the biotechnology industry). The only recommended workplace exposure limit for a product of biotechnology is for subtilisins: ACGIH's ceiling threshold limit value (TLV) is 0.00006 mg/m^3 (60 ng/m^3) for a 60-min sample.[9]

OSHA's bloodborne pathogens standard (29 CFR 1910.1030) requires that HBV vaccinations be made available to those occupationally exposed, and that post-exposure evaluations and follow-up be conducted in the event of a significant exposure to blood or other potentially infectious materials.[10] But the standard does not mandate medical surveillance of workers potentially exposed to bloodborne pathogens.

The NIH *Guidelines for Research Involving Recombinant DNA Molecules* impose a responsibility on institutions performing recombinant DNA work within the scope of the guidelines to "determine the necessity for health surveillance of recombinant DNA research personnel, and conduct, if found appropriate, a health surveillance program . . ."[1] The program elements suggested in the NIH Guidelines are:

- records of agents handled;
- active investigations of relevant illnesses; and
- maintenance of serial serum samples for monitoring serologic changes that may result from employee work experience.

If agents that require BSL3 or greater physical containment are to be handled, the NIH Guidelines require collection and storage of baseline serum samples and collection of additional serum samples if the agents handled warrant them. A health surveillance program is required by the guidelines only if personnel are engaged in large-scale work with agents that require BSL3 or greater containment. This program is to include at a minimum:

- preassignment and periodic physical and medical examinations;
- collection, maintenance, and analysis of serum specimens for monitoring work-related serologic changes; and
- provisions for the investigation of any serious, unusual, or extended employee illnesses possibly related to work.

Examples listed in the guidelines of medical conditions that might place a worker at increased risk of work-related illness and, thereby, preclude his or her involvement in a project are:

- gastrointestinal disorders, which could reduce the employee's resistance to coliform or other enteropathogenic microorganisms; and
- treatment with steroids, immunosuppressive drugs, or antibiotics, which could reduce the employee's immunological competence.

The NIH Guidelines also impose on the institution, the Institutional Biosafety Committee, the Biological Safety Officer, and the Principal Investigator the responsibility to "report significant research-related illnesses. . ." and require that if a research group is working with a known pathogen for which there is an effective vaccine, the vaccine should be made available.

The CDC/NIOSH Ad Hoc Working Group on Medical Surveillance for Industrial Application of Biotechnology was convened to develop additional guidance to institutions on medical surveillance of biotechnology workers. The working group concluded that:[6]

- Industrial applications of biotechnologies will increase the potential for worker exposure to rDNA microorganisms and products.
- The health hazards of the current commonly used strains seem minimal.
- The health hazards of the products of these organisms seem to be more substantial.
- Medical surveillance programs should be highly specific: they should be designed to evaluate the specific hazards that confront an occupational group; and

- Establishment of medical surveillance in any newly developed industry constitutes prudent medical practice.

These conclusions and recommendations are shared by the "Specialist Working Group on Health Surveillance of Those Involved in Genetic Manipulation at Laboratory and Large Scale" of the Advisory Committee on Genetic Manipulation of Britain's Health and Safety Executive.[11] According to the advisory statements of this committee and the CDC/NIOSH working group — and most authors on the subject — the guiding principle when designing a medical surveillance program for workers potentially exposed to biohazards is that the program elements should be targeted to the foreseeable consequences of exposure to the agents handled.[4,12]

In summary, medical surveillance should occupy a central role in the health and safety program of a biomedical research or biotechnology facility. Because of the difficulties in applying traditional industrial hygiene exposure assessment techniques to biohazards, one relies on medical surveillance to detect exposure and occupational illness. The process by which a medical surveillance program is developed should be identical to that followed in other industries. The elements of the medical surveillance program and the timing of the examinations should be selected based on the anticipated health effects of the agents handled by the exposure group.

3.   Transportation and Shipping of Biological Materials *

Background

In general, interstate transportation of biohazardous materials is subject to U.S. Public Health Service (PHS) and Department of Transportation (DOT) regulations. The DOT and PHS govern interstate transportation by rail, air, vessel, and public highway. The regulations of the International Air Transport Association (IATA) and the International Civil Aviation Organization (ICAO) also apply when biohazardous materials are shipped by air. All biohazardous materials leaving facilities must meet all applicable requirements. The employee who uses a commercial carrier or personally carries a package in his or her own car, a company vehicle, taxi, or bus is responsible for ensuring that all legal requirements are met for packaging, labeling, and documentation. **The type of packaging, labeling, and documentation required depends on the type of biohazardous material being shipped and how it is to be shipped (i.e., the mode of transportation and the temperature requirements of the materials).** DOT, PHS, and IATA/ICAO packaging and labeling requirements are given below.

Some institutions require that a Principal Investigator preapprove transfer of materials under his or her direction. Biohazardous materials moved between buildings of the same facility are not subject to DOT regulations when travel over public roads is not involved. Biosafety principles, however, require that these biohazardous materials be transported in durable, leakproof, labeled containers.

Further Classification of Biohazardous Materials

DOT definition: An *infectious substance* means a viable microorganism, or its toxin, that causes or might cause disease in humans or animals, and includes those agents listed in 42 CFR 72.3 of U.S. Department of Health and Human Services (DHHS) regulations or any other agent that causes or might cause severe disabling or fatal disease. Infectious substance and etiologic agent are synonymous. [This definition is consistent with that of the PHS.]

IATA/ICAO definition: An *infectious substance* contains viable microorganisms including a bacterium, virus, rickettsia, parasite, fungus, or a recombinant,hybrid or mutant, that are known or reasonably believed to cause disease in humans or animals. Infectious substances are further classified into four risk groups, with IV being high individual and community risk and I being low individual and community risk. Infectious substances in risk group I are not subject to IATA (ICAO) regulations.

DOT and PHS definitions: A *diagnostic specimen* means any human or animal material including, but not limited to, excreta, secreta, blood and its components, tissue, and tissue fluids being shipped for the purpose of diagnosis.

---

* Adapted from 49 CFR Parts 100-199; *Dangerous Goods Regulations,* 36th Edition, International Air Transport Association, Geneva, Switzerland, 1995; and "Guidelines for Research Involving Recombinant DNA Molecules (NIH Guidelines)," *Federal Register 59:*127 (5 July 1994). pp. 34496-34547.

IATA/ICAO definition: A *diagnostic specimen* means any human or animal material including, but not limited to, excreta, secreta, blood and its components, tissue, and tissue fluids being shipped for the purpose of diagnosis, excluding live infected animals. Diagnostic specimens are further classified by IATA/ICAO into three categories that require different packaging. One category consists of those being transported to undergo confirmatory testing. These are known to contain or believed likely to contain infectious substances. The second category consists of those diagnostic specimens being transported to undergo routine screening tests or for the purpose of initial diagnosis. These are considered to involve a relatively low probability that infectious substances are present. The third category includes diagnostic specimens that are known *not* to contain infectious substances. This category is not restricted by IATA/ICAO. It must be noted, however, that knowledge that a diagnostic specimen is free of infectious substances necessarily requires extensive testing or knowledge of treatment.

NOTE: Transportation of diagnostic specimens is not regulated by the DOT. Note, however, that if ground or vessel transportation of diagnostic specimens is required *prior to* air transportation, the DOT requires that IATA/ICAO requirements be met (49 CFR 171.11-171.12).

A *biological product* means a material prepared and manufactured in accordance with the provisions of the following and which may be shipped in interstate commerce:

- 9 CFR Part 102: Licenses for biological products
- 9 CFR Part 103: Biological products for experimental treatment of animals
- 9 CFR Part 104: Permits for biological products
- 21 CFR Part 312: Investigational new drug application
- 21 CFR Parts 600–680: Biologics

Requirements for biological products will not be presented here.

Packaging of Infectious Substances

DOT packaging requirements for infectious substances:

- Packaging of infectious substances requires inner packagings and an outer packaging. The inner packagings consist of a watertight primary receptacle, a watertight secondary packaging, and an absorbent material placed between the primary receptacle and secondary packaging. If multiple-primary receptacles are placed in a single secondary packaging, they must be wrapped individually to ensure that contact between them is prevented. The absorbent material (such as cotton wool) must be sufficient to absorb the entire contents of all primary receptacles. The outer packaging must be of adequate strength for the package's capacity, mass, and intended use.
- Each package for infectious substances must be capable of passing the tests specified by the DOT (49 CFR 178.609). Packages consigned as freight must be at least 100 mm (3.9 in.) in the smallest overall external dimension. All primary receptacles *and* secondary packaging used for infectious substances must be capable of withstanding, without leakage, an internal pressure that produces a pressure differential of not less than 95 kPa (14 psi) and temperatures in the range of -40°C to +55°C (-40°F to +131°F).
- The primary receptacle of *lyophilized substances* include flame-sealed glass ampoules or rubber-stoppered glass vials with fitted metal seals.
- Appropriate packaging of liquid or solid substances depends on the temperature at which they are shipped and the volume or mass.

The following apply for volumes greater than or equal to 50 mL:

- For those shipped at ambient or higher temperatures, primary receptacles include those of glass, metal, or plastic. Positive means of ensuring a leakproof seal (such as heat seal, skirted stopper, or metal crimp seal) must be provided. If screw caps are used, they must be reinforced with adhesive tape.
- For *liquid or solid substances shipped at refrigerated temperatures or frozen (including ice, prefrozen packs, and dry ice)* ice or dry ice must be placed outside the secondary packaging. Interior supports must be provided to secure the secondary packaging in the original position after the ice or dry ice has dissipated. If ice is used, the packaging must be leakproof. If dry ice is used, the outer packaging must allow for the release of carbon dioxide gas.

- For *liquid or solid substances shipped in liquid nitrogen,* primary receptacles capable of withstanding very low temperatures must be used. Secondary packaging must also withstand very low temperatures and will need to be fitted over individual primary receptacles in most cases. Requirements for shipping liquid nitrogen must also be observed.

All requirements for ≤ 50 mL, plus the following, apply for volumes > 50 mL:

- Shock-absorbent material, in a volume at least equal to that of the absorbent material between the primary and secondary containers, shall be placed at the top, bottom, and sides between the secondary container and the outer shipping container. Single primary containers shall not contain more than 1 L of material; however, two or more primary containers whose combined volumes does not exceed 1 L may be placed in a single, secondary container. The maximum amount of etiologic agent that may be enclosed within a single outer shipping container must not exceed 4 L.
- DOT requirements limit the quantity of infectious substances to 50 mL (liquid) or 50 g (solid) for passenger aircraft or railcar and 4 L (liquid) or 4 kg (solid) for cargo aircraft.

IATA/ICAO packaging requirements for infectious substances:

Following is the one IATA/ICAO "packaging instruction" for infectious substances (602):

- Packaging of infectious substances requires inner packagings and an outer packaging. The inner packagings consist of a watertight primary receptacle, a watertight secondary packaging, and an absorbent material placed between the primary receptacle and secondary packaging. If multiple primary receptacles are placed in a single secondary packaging, they must be wrapped individually to ensure that contact between them is prevented. The absorbent material (such as cotton wool) must be sufficient to absorb the entire contents of all primary receptacles. The outer packaging must be of sufficient strength to meet the design type tests found in Subsection 10.5 of the IATA 1995 regulations.
- Packages consigned as freight must be at least 100 mm (3.9 in.) in the smallest overall external dimension.
- An itemized list of contents must be enclosed between the secondary packaging and the outer packaging.
- All primary receptacles **OR** the secondary packaging used for infectious substances must be capable of withstanding, without leakage, an internal pressure that produces a pressure differential of not less than 95 kPa (14 psi) and temperatures in the range of -40°C to +55°C (-40°F to +131°F).
- All packages must be marked durably and legibly on the outside of the package with the name and telephone number of a person responsible for the shipment.

Also, the following specific requirements must be met for temperatures at which infectious substances must be shipped:

- For infectious substances *shipped at ambient temperatures or higher,* primary receptacles may only be of glass, metal, or plastic. A positive means of ensuring a leakproof seal must be provided (such as heat seal, skirted stopper, or metal crimp seal). If screw caps are used, they must be reinforced with adhesive tape.
- For infectious substances *shipped refrigerated or frozen (wet ice, prefrozen packs, dry ice),* the ice or dry ice must be placed outside the secondary packaging(s). Interior support must be provided to secure the secondary packaging(s) in the original position after the ice or dry ice has dissipated. If ice is used, the packaging must be leakproof. If dry ice is used, the outer packaging must allow for the release of carbon dioxide gas. The primary receptacle and the secondary packaging must maintain their containment integrity at the temperature of the refrigerant used as well as at the temperatures and pressure(s) of air transport to which the receptacle could be subjected if refrigeration were to be lost.
- For infectious substances *shipped in liquid nitrogen,* plastic primary receptacles capable of withstanding very low temperatures must be used. Secondary packaging must also withstand very low temperatures and in most cases will need to be fitted over individual primary receptacles. Requirements for shipment of liquid nitrogen must also be observed. The primary receptacle must maintain its containment integrity at the temperature of the refrigerant used as well as at the tempera-

tures and pressure(s) of air transport to which the receptacle could be subjected if refrigeration were to be lost.
- For shipping *lyophilized infectious substances,* primary receptacles must be either flame-sealed glass ampoules or rubber-stoppered glass vials with metal seals.
- Quantity restrictions apply. No more than 50 mL (liquid) or 50 g (solid) net quantity per package can be shipped on passenger aircraft. No more than 4 L (liquid) or 4 kg (solid) net quantity per package can be shipped on cargo aircraft.

PHS packaging requirements for infectious substances:

The PHS regulations for the interstate shipping of infectious agents are being revised, but the following requirements were in effect at publication of this manual. These requirements apply to certain infectious agents that are listed by PHS; however, because this list does not contain all of the infectious agents that PHS wishes to regulate, it is under revision. Also, some infectious agents must be sent by registered mail or an equivalent system.

- *Volumes ≤ 50 mL:* Infectious material must be placed in a secure, watertight primary container (e.g., test tube, vial) that must be enclosed in a second, durable watertight secondary container. Several primary containers may be enclosed in a single secondary container, if the total volume of all primary containers does not exceed 50 mL. All space between the primary and secondary containers shall contain sufficient absorbent material to absorb the entire contents of the primary container(s) in case of breakage or leakage. Each set of primary and secondary containers must then be enclosed in an outer shipping container constructed of corrugated fiberboard, cardboard, wood, or other material of equivalent strength.
- *Volumes > 50 mL:* All requirements for volumes ≤ 50 mL (listed above) must be met. Also, a shock-absorbent material, in volume at least equal to that of the absorbent material between the primary and secondary containers, must be placed in all spaces between the secondary container and the outer shipping container. Single primary containers whose combined volumes do not exceed 1 L may be placed in a single, secondary container. The maximum volume that may be enclosed in a single outer shipping container cannot exceed 4 L.
- If dry ice is used as a refrigerant, it must be placed outside the secondary container(s). If dry ice is used between the secondary container and the outer shipping container, the outer container must allow for the release of carbon dioxide gas.

Packaging Requirements for Diagnostic Specimens

There are no DOT requirements for packaging diagnostic specimens, but following are IATA/ICAO packaging requirements for diagnostic specimens:

- For shipping diagnostic specimens known to contain or believed likely to contain infectious substances, follow the IATA/ICAO requirements above (i.e., use "packaging instruction" 602).
- For diagnostic specimens known not to contain infectious substances, there are no IATA/ICAO requirements.
- For diagnostic specimens with a low probability of containing infectious substances, "packaging instruction" 650 must be used. The requirements follow:
  - Inner packagings must consist of a leakproof primary receptacle(s), a watertight secondary packaging, an absorbent material, and an outer packaging of adequate strength for its capacity, weight, and intended use. Absorbent material must be placed between the primary receptacle and the secondary packaging. If multiple primary receptacles are placed in a single secondary packaging, they must be wrapped individually to ensure that contact between them is prevented. The absorbing material (such as cotton wool) must be sufficient to absorb the entire contents of all primary receptacles.
  - The entire package must be capable of withstanding at least a 1.2 m drop test on a hard unyielding surface without release of its contents. The primary receptacle **OR** the secondary packaging used for biological products and diagnostic specimens must be capable of withstanding, without leakage, an internal pressure that produces a pressure differential of not less than 95 kPa in the range of -40°C to +55°C (-40°F to 131°F).

- Packages consigned as freight must be at least 100 mm (3.9 in) in the smallest overall external dimension.
  - Also, specific requirements for temperatures at which infectious substances must be shipped also apply to diagnostic specimens with a relatively low probability of the presence of infectious substances.

PHS packaging requirements for diagnostic specimens:

The PHS regulations for the interstate shipping of infectious agents and diagnostic specimens are being revised. PHS currently requires that diagnostic specimens with a low probability of containing infectious agents meet IATA/ICAO "packaging instruction" 650.

Labeling of Packagings of Infectious Substances and Diagnostic Specimens

DOT labeling requirements are as follows:

- The DOT Infectious Substance label is required for both intrastate and interstate shipping destinations. It has a white background with *Infectious Substance* in black lettering.
- The DOT does not regulate the transportation of diagnostic specimens; therefore, there are no DOT labeling requirements.

IATA/ICAO labeling requirements are as follows:

The Infectious Substance label is required for infectious substances and for diagnostic specimens known to contain infectious substances. The label is diamond-shaped (with square dimensions 100 × 100 mm, minimum) with specific markings. The universal biohazard symbol is pictured in black in the top corner and the lower part of the label bears the following inscription in black lettering: INFECTIOUS SUBSTANCE — IN CASE OF DAMAGE OR LEAKAGE IMMEDIATELY NOTIFY PUBLIC HEALTH AUTHORITY. The background of the label is white.

For small packages, the dimensions of these labels may be no smaller than 50 × 50 mm.

Labeling is not required for diagnostic specimens either known not to contain infectious substances or for those with a low probability of containing infectious substances.

PHS labeling requirements are as follows:

The PHS label for infectious substances and diagnostic specimens is identical. It has the following aspects: a rectangle measuring 51 mm (2 in.) by 102.5 mm (4 in.), a red universal biohazard symbol on a white background, and lettering in both red and white, and the following inscription: ETIOLOGIC AGENTS — BIOMEDICAL MATERIAL — IN CASE OF DAMAGE OR LEAKAGE NOTIFY DIRECTOR CDC ATLANTA, GEORGIA 404-633-5313.

Documentation

An itemized list of contents must be enclosed between the secondary packaging and the outer packaging. An exact description of the contents of primary receptacles for the shipping manifest must be provided to personnel who actually ship the material. This information is necessary so that personnel can accurately fill out additional paperwork and mark the outer packages appropriately.

4. Use of Laboratory Equipment

Pipets are basic scientific pieces of equipment used throughout the world. They are used for volumetric measurement of fluids and for the transfer of these fluids from one container to another. The fluids that are handled are frequently hazardous in nature, containing infectious, toxic, corrosive or radioactive agents. A pipet can become a hazardous piece of equipment if used improperly. Safety pipetting techniques are required to reduce the potential for exposure to hazardous materials. The most common hazards associated with pipetting procedures involve the application of mouth suction. The causative event in more than 13% of all known laboratory accidents that resulted in infection was oral aspiration through a pipet. Contaminants can be transferred to the mouth if a contaminated finger is placed on the suction end of the pipet. There is also the danger of inhaling aerosols created in the handling of liquid suspensions when using unplugged pipets, even if no liquid is drawn into the mouth.

Other hazards of exposure to aerosols are created by liquid dropping from a pipet to a work surface, by mixing cultures by alternate suction and blowing, by forceful ejection of an inoculum onto a culture dish, or by blowing out the last drop. It has been demonstrated by high-speed photography that an aerosol of approximately 15,000 droplets — most under 10 μm — is produced when the last drop of fluid in the tip of the pipet is blown out with moderate force. Although the aerosol hazard associated with pipetting procedures can be reduced only by use of safe techniques and biological safety cabinets, the potential hazards associated with oral ingestion can be eliminated by use of mechanical pipetting aids.

Safe Practices Governing the Use of Pipets and Pipetting Aids *

1. Never use mouth pipetting. Always use some type of pipetting aid.
2. If working with biohazardous or toxic fluids, pipetting operations should be confined to a safety cabinet or hood.
3. Pipets used for the pipetting of biohazardous or toxic materials always should be plugged with cotton (even when safety pipetting aids are used).
4. No biohazardous material should be prepared by bubbling expiratory air through a liquid with a pipet.
5. Biohazardous material should not be mixed by suction and expulsion through a pipet.
6. No biohazardous material should be forcibly expelled out of a pipet.
7. When pipets are used, avoid accidentally dropping infectious cultures from the pipet. Place a disinfectant-soaked towel on the working surface and autoclave the towel after use.
8. Transfer of liquid between the graduation marks of pipets is preferable to expelling the last drop.
9. Discharge from pipets should be as close as possible to the fluid or agar level, or the contents should be allowed to run down the wall of the tube or bottle whenever possible, not dropped from a height.
10. Nondisposable pipets contaminated with potentially infectious material should be placed horizontally in a pan containing enough suitable disinfectant to allow complete immersion. They should not be placed vertically in a cylinder.
11. Discard pans for used pipets are to be housed within the biological safety cabinet.
12. The pan and pipets should be autoclaved as a unit. The replacement unit should be a clean pan with fresh disinfectant.

5. Housekeeping **

Housekeeping procedures and schedules are essential in limiting exposure to biohazardous materials. The objectives of housekeeping in the biological laboratory are to:

- provide an orderly and clean work area conducive to the accomplishment of the research program;
- provide work areas devoid of physical hazards;
- prevent the accumulation of materials from current and past experiments that constitute hazard to laboratory personnel; and
- prevent the creation of aerosols of hazardous materials as a result of the housekeeping procedures used.

The primary function of routine housekeeping procedures is to prevent the accumulation of wastes that 1) might harbor microorganisms that are a threat to the integrity of the biological systems under investigation; 2) might enhance the survival of microorganisms inadvertently released in experimental procedures; 3) might retard penetration of disinfectants; 4) might be transferable from one area to another on clothing and shoes; 5) might, with sufficient buildup, become a biohazard as a consequence of secondary aerosolization by personnel and air movement; and 6) might cause allergic sensitization of personnel (e.g., to animal dander).

---

* Adapted from *Laboratory Safety Monograph — A Supplement to the NIH Guidelines for Recombinant DNA Research,* USDHEW, USPHS, NIH, January 1979.

** Adapted from *Laboratory Safety Monograph — A Supplement to the NIH Guidelines for Recombinant DNA Research,* USDHEW, USPHS, NIH, July 1978.

Housekeeping in animal care units has the same primary function as that described for the laboratory and should also be carried out as meticulously in quarantine and conditioning areas as in areas used to house experimentally infected animals. No other areas in the laboratory have the constant potential for creation of significant quantities of contaminated waste than animal care facilities.

Floor Care: Avoidance of dry sweeping and dusting will reduce the formation of nonspecific environmental aerosols. Wet mopping or vacuum cleaning with a high-efficiency particulate air (HEPA) filter on the exhaust is recommended.

In the absence of overt hazardous spills, the cleaning process commonly will consist of an initial vacuuming to remove all gross particulate matter and a follow-up wet mopping with a solution of chemical decontaminant containing a detergent. Depending on the nature of the surfaces to be cleaned and the availability of floor drains, removal of residual cleaning solutions can be accomplished by a number of methods. Among these are pickup with a partially dry mop, pickup with a wet vacuum that has an adequately filtered exhaust, or removal to an convenient floor drain by use of a floor squeegee.

Dry Sweeping: Although it is recommended that dry sweeping be minimized as much as possible, this might be the only method available or practicable under certain circumstances. In such cases, sweeping compounds used with push brooms and dry-dust mopheads treated to suppress aerosolization of dust should be used.

D. Engineering Controls

Safety equipment includes biological safety cabinets and a variety of enclosed containers. Safety equipment also includes items for personal protection such as gloves, coats, gowns, shoe covers, boots, respirators, face shields, and safety glasses. These personal protective devices are often used in combination with biological safety cabinets and other devices that contain the agents, animals, or materials being worked with. In some situations, however, it is impractical to work in biological safety cabinets, meaning personal protective devices may form the primary barrier between personnel and the infectious materials. Certain animal studies, animal necropsy, production activities, and activities relating to maintenance, service, or support of the laboratory facility are examples of these situations.

A comprehensive safety program for a research facility using biological agents can be developed by using a strategy of primary and secondary containment. Primary containment is the protection of personnel and the immediate laboratoryor production environment. It is provided by good microbiological techniques and the use of appropriate safety equipment. Secondary containment is the protection of the environment external to the laboratory from exposure to infectious materials. It is provided by a combination of facility design and operational practices.

1.   Primary Barriers *

Engineering controls normally consist of primary and secondary barriers. Primary barriers help safeguard laboratory personnel from hazardous research materials; secondary barriers help the environment. Also, some of these systems have been effective in maintaining the purity of research materials. Contamination detrimental to the research mission may include ubiquitous fungal or bacterial contamination from outdoors, indoors, equipment, or even laboratory personnel. The potential for cross-contamination of research materials within the facility also can be reduced by barrier systems.

A primary barrier is interposed between the agent and the personnel. A primary barrier is intended to confine and isolate the agent from the individual manipulating the agent and provide protection to other persons in the laboratory room. Primary barriers can be designed to enclose simple manipulations (e.g., pipetting) or complex processes such as continuous-flow centrifugation.

Primary barriers generally are represented by biological safety cabinets, laboratory fume hoods, and glove boxes. These systems are manufactured by assembling in various combinations and configurations:

- Physical barriers (impervious surfaces such as metal sides, glass panels, rubber gloves, and gaskets);
- Air barriers (flow of air with relatively uniform direction and velocity);

---

* Adapted from *Design of Biomedical Research Facilities, Cancer Research Safety Monograph, Vol. 4* (NIH Publication No. 81-2305), USDHHS, USPHS, NIH, 1981.

- Filtration barriers (HEPA filters); and
- Inactivation or destruction barriers (autoclaves and incinerators).

Biological Safety Cabinets

Several models of cabinets with varied containment capabilities have been marketed throughout the years. Three primary classes of biological safety cabinets (Class I, II, and III) have now become widely recognized. Each class is distinguished by its design and its containment and cleanliness capability. Class I and Class II cabinets have an air barrier between the laboratory operator and the cabinet work area. Since air barriers do not provide absolute containment, these two classes of cabinets are considered to be partial containment devices. Class III cabinets have physical barriers between the operator and the cabinet work area and are considered "absolute" containment devices. NIH formalized recommended performance specifications for all three classes of cabinets in its *Laboratory Safety Monograph,* published in 1979. These appear in Table XX.

Table XX. Recommended Minimum Performance Specifications of Biological Safety Cabinets

Cabinet	Face Velocity (ft/min)	Velocity Profile	Negative Pressure (inches, w.g.)	Permissible Leak Rate [A]	Exhaust Filter Efficiency
Class I:					
Open front	75	N/A	N/A	N/A	99.97% for 0.3 µm particles
Front panel without gloves	150	N/A	N/A	N/A	"
Front panel with gloves	N/A	N/A	p 0.5	N/A	"
Class II:					
Type A	75	[B]	N/A	1×10^{-4} cc/sec at 2 in. w.g. pressure [C]	"
Type B	100	[B]	N/A	N/A	"
100% Exhaust	100	[B]	N/A	N/A	"
Class III:					
	N/A	N/A	p 0.5	1×10^{-5} cc/sec at 3 in. w.g. pressure	[D]

N/A = not applicable

[A] This leak rate refers to the carcus of the cabinet.

[B] Depends on National Sanitation Foundation (NSF) certification in accordance with NSF Standard 49.

[C] For biologically contaminated positive-pressure plenums.

[D] Both HEPA filters must be certified to have a filtration efficiency of 99.97% for 0.3 µm particles. When an incinerator is used in lieu of the second HEPA filter, the incinerator must be capable of destroying all spores of *Bacillus subtilis* when challenged at a concentration of 10^5 spores per cubic foot of air.

The **Class I** cabinet is a conventional, open-face, negative-pressure cabinet similar in concept to a laboratory fume hood (see Figure 3). These cabinets provide personnel and environmental protection and are suitable for BSL1, BSL2, and BSL3 containment.

Class II cabinets, commonly known as laminar flow biological safety cabinets, were developed to protect the operator from research materials and to protect the research materials from external contamination. HEPA-filtered air flows from an overhead diffuser down over the work area, providing a contamination-free zone. This downflow air splits at the work surface, with part flowing to a grille at the rear of the work surface and part flowing to a grille at the front (see Figures 4, 5, and 6). Operators are

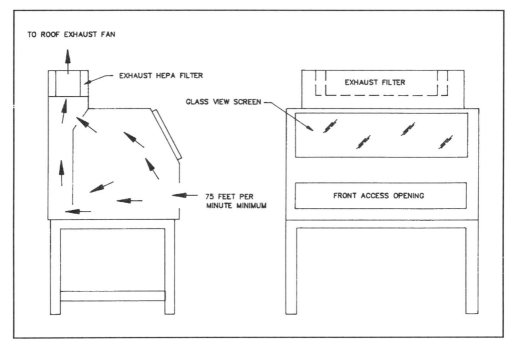

Figure 3. Class I biological safety cabinet.

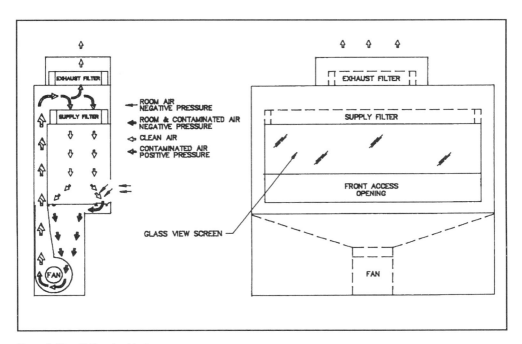

Figure 4. Class II, Type A cabinet.

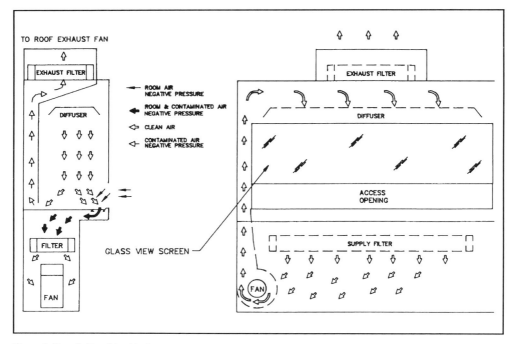

Figure 5. Class II, Type B1 cabinet.

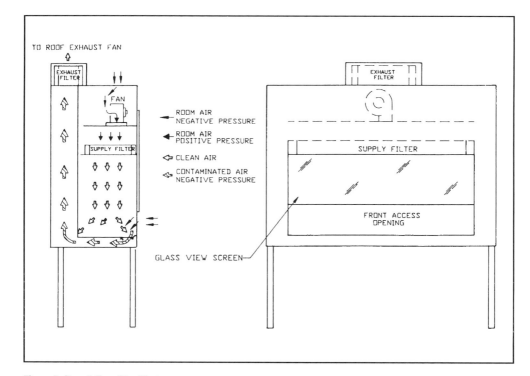

Figure 6. Class II, Type B2 cabinet.

protected by the air barrier created by the inflow of room air and the downflow air that flows into the front grille.

There are three basic types of Class II cabinets: Type A (Figure 4), formerly known as Type 1; Type B1 (Figure 5), formerly known as Type 2, and Type B2 (Figure 6), sometimes referred to as 100% exhaust; and Type B3. These types differ in the proportion of air recirculated into the work area; the velocities of the airflows into the work opening and downward to the work surface; the manner of discharge of exhaust air; and the pressure in contaminated air plenums relative to the room.

Features of the Class II, Type A (also known as NSF A) cabinet:

- The optimum work opening is generally 8 in. (0.2 m) in height. A 10-in. (0.25-m) work opening height is sometimes used.
- Approximately 70% of the total air moved is recirculated into the work area from a common plenum. Approximately 30% of the total air comes into the cabinet through the work opening; an amount equal to the intake is discharged through the exhaust outlet.
- The intake velocity at the work opening has at least 75 ft/min (0.38 m/sec.); the vertical flow downward toward the work surface varies with design.
- A blower, an integral part of the cabinet, forces portions of the contaminated air drawn from the work area through the supply (recirculation) filter and the exhaust filter; thus, exhaust air is forcefully discharged by the cabinet.
- The contaminated air plenum between the blower and the filters is under positive pressure. In some designs, this plenum is at positive pressure to the room and has to be gas-tight. In other patented designs, it is surrounded by plenums at negative pressure to the room.
- The sash may be fixed, hinged, or sliding.
- The Type A cabinet will operate free-standing with HEPA-filtered exhaust air dumping back into the room.

Features of the Class II, Type B (NSF B1) cabinet:

- It has a movable sash that can be raised from the usual work opening of 8 in. (0.2 m) to 20 in. (0.5 m) for introduction and removal of equipment and materials.
- From 30% to 50% of the air is recirculated in the cabinet. The balance (50% to 70%) of the air comes into the cabinet through the work opening; an equal amount is drawn out through the exhaust outlet.
- The intake air velocity at the work opening is a minimum of 100 ft/min (0.5 m/sec.) at the normal working opening of 8 in.; the vertical flow downward toward the work surface varies with design.
- A blower or blowers in the base of the cabinet draw air through a grille near the work opening and then through a supply HEPA filter. The blowers force filtered air up through plenums along the sides of the cabinet and downward through an overhead diffuser above the work surface. Some cabinets now have a second supply filter directly above the work area. Air is drawn from the work area through a rear grille and via a dedicated plenum through a HEPA filter by an exhaust blower that is usually located on the roof of the building. Thus, exhaust air must be drawn from the cabinet by an external fan, and the air recirculated to the work area is never mixed with air that is being exhausted.
- The contaminated air plenums are at negative pressure relative to the room.
- A building blower and duct system is required for the cabinet to operate.

Features of the Class II, 100% (NSF B2) exhaust cabinet:

- It has a movable sash similar to the Type B cabinet.
- No air is recirculated to the work area; 100% of the air moved in the cabinet is directly exhausted from the work area.
- A supply blower forces air from outside the cabinet through a supply HEPA filter and down through the work area.
- An exhaust blower on the roof of the building draws air into the cabinet through the work opening. It then pulls all of this intake air, plus all of the air that was supplied to the top of the work area, through a HEPA filter and exhausts it to the outside of the building.
- A building blower and duct system is required for the cabinet to operate.

Features of the NSF B3 cabinet:

- This is a Class II, Type A cabinet with three conditions applied:
  - minimum of 100 fpm intake air velocity;
  - no biologically contaminated plenums positive to the room; and
  - air exhausted from the cabinet is ducted to the outdoors.

Class III cabinets are hermetically sealed enclosures for confining extremely hazardous materials. Operators must perform their work by inserting their hands and arms into long rubber gloves attached to the cabinet, which serve as physical barriers (see Figure 7). For this, gloves made of neoprene in thicknesses of 15 to 30 mil have been found to be satisfactory; however, they must be inspected for pinhole leaks as received from the manufacturer and at routine intervals of use. Some manufacturers will give assurance that their gloves have been tested by resistance to high voltage as evidence they are free of thin areas and pinholes. After intervals of service, and after sterilization of the cabinet system, the gloves — while still attached to the cabinets — should be examined for leaks using halogen at 3 inches water column (in. w.c.) following the certification procedures for Class III cabinet systems. There will be no further discussion of Class III cabinets since they are used only in maximum containment facilities.

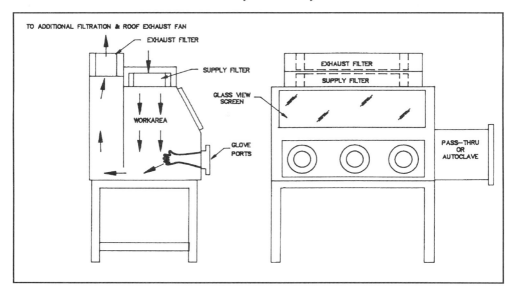

Figure 7. Class III cabinet.

Inherent in the features of these biological safety cabinets are certain assets and limitations. These features must be understood so that proper consideration of the assets and limitations can be made when selecting the cabinets and designing their installation (see Table XXI).

Table XXI. Applications of Biological Safety Cabinets in Microbiological Research

	Biological Safety Cabinet			Research Uses/Applications		
Type	Work Opening		Face Velocity (ft/min)	Oncogenic Viruses [A]	Chemical Carcinogens [B]	Etiologic Agents [C]/ Recombinant DNA [D]
Class I:						
	Front panel not in place		75	Low and moderate	No	BSL3
	Front panel in place without gloves		150	Low and moderate	Yes	BSL3

	Front panel in place with gloves	N/A	Low and moderate	Yes	BSL3
Class II:					
Type A (NSF-A)	Fixed height, usually 10 in.	75 min	Low and moderate	No	BSL3
Type B and 100% Exhaust (NSF B1, B2, and B3)	Sliding sash provides opening adjustable from 8 to 30 in. for introduction and removal of equipment and materials. To obtain proper face velocity, experimentation should be done with 8-in. opening.	100 at 8-in. opening	Low and moderate	Yes, in low dilution and volatility	BSL3
Class III:	No direct opening. Access is through double-door sterilizer and decontaminant dunk bath.	N/A	Low, moderate, and high	Yes	BSL4

A **U.S. Department of Health, Education and Welfare, National Cancer Institute, Office of Research Safety:** *Safety Standards for Research Involving Oncogenic Viruses* (DHEW Publication No. [NIH] 78-790. Bethesda, Md: National Cancer Institute, 1978.

B **U.S. Department of Health, Education and Welfare, National Cancer Institute, Office of Research Safety:** *Safety Standards for Research Involving Chemical Carcinogens* (DHEW Publication No. [NIH] 76-900). Bethesda, Md.: National Cancer Institute,*U.S. Department of Health, Education and Welfare*, 1976.

C **U.S. Department of Health, Education and Welfare, Public Health Services, Centers for Disease Control and Prevention:** *Classification of Etiologic Agents on the Basis of Hazard.* Atlanta, Ga.: Centers for Disease Control, 1974.

D **U.S. Department of Health, Education and Welfare, National Institutes of Health:** *National Institutes of Health Safety Monograph* (A Supplement to the NIH Guidelines for Recombinant DNA Research). Bethesda, Md.: National Institutes of Health, 1978.

Some of these assets and limitations are discussed quantitatively in the literature.[13-15]

Design Considerations for Installing Biological Safety Cabinets

Requirements for the proper installation of a biological safety cabinet depend on the class of cabinet and on the nature of the research and the materials to be handled. Considerations must also be made for the safety of maintenance personnel who will service the mechanical equipment. Design considerations for the maintenance of laboratory facilities must be considered. Aside from maintenance, the design engineer must consider the following:

a. *Location of the cabinet within the room:* Extraneous air currents near the work opening of a cabinet can disrupt the inward airflow and jeopardize containment and product protection. These air currents can be caused by the swinging motion of nearby doors, personnel walking past the front of the cabinet, or drafts from ventilation outlets. Cabinets therefore should be located out of traffic patterns and away from doors, preferably at the "dead-end" of the laboratory. The discharge from nearby ventilation outlets should be directed away from the cabinets.

b. *Cabinet exhaust system:* The exhaust system should have provisions for decontamination such as an air tight dampener.

Class I: HEPA-filtered air sometimes may be returned to the laboratory environment, provided 1) that the exhaust filter has been certified, and 2) that use of volatile, toxic, or radioactive materials in the cabinet is prohibited. Note that the Class I cabinet usually does not have an integral blower and an air mover remotely located must be provided. Class I cabinets are usually connected directly to an exhaust system that discharges to the outdoors.

Class II, Type A: This type of cabinet has an integral exhaust blower and the HEPA-filtered air may be discharged to the room, provided 1) that the exhaust filter has been certified; 2) that the use of volatile, toxic, or radioactive materials in the cabinet is prohibited; and 3) there is adequate clearance to the ceiling so that exhaust air is not restricted. In this case, a guard to protect the exhaust HEPA filter from damage should be installed. It is preferable, however, to discharge the exhaust air outdoors. An air mover remotely located must be provided to take the air from the top of the cabinet and discharge it outside. A hard connection or a thimble connection may be used at the top of the cabinet.

   Class II, Type B and 100% exhaust: These types of cabinets require an external exhaust blower and must be hard connected directly to an exhaust system that discharges to the outdoors.

    c. *Use of toxic chemicals and chemical carcinogens:* Many laboratories (e.g., virology and cell culture laboratories) use dilute preparations of chemical carcinogens and other toxic substances. The likelihood of the use of carcinogens or toxic chemicals in your laboratory should be evaluated before selecting and installing biological safety cabinets. Careful evaluation must be made of problems for decontaminating the cabinet and associated exhaust system (prior to maintenance activity). Air purification systems such as charcoal filter beds, catalytic converters, and incinerators may be required for the cabinet effluents to meet any applicable emission regulations.

    d. *Quantities of supply and exhaust air:* The quantity of air exhausted through a properly operating laboratory fume hood or biological safety cabinet must be known when designing the air balance for the facility. Approximate values of required make-up air are given in Table XXII. Required face velocities (and thus the requirements for make-up air) for Class I cabinets and laboratory fume hoods may vary with application, but operating specifications for Class II cabinets (types A and B) are firmly established: The air quantities for these cabinets must always be within ± 5% of the manufacturer's specified values. Otherwise, the operator or product protection could be jeopardized.

Table XXII. Make-Up Air Requirements for Laboratory Hoods and Safety Cabinets

Type of Hood or Cabinet	Minimum Average Face Velocity (ft/min)	Approximate Make-Up Air Requirements (ft^3/min)	
		4-ft Hood	6-ft Hood
Class I:	75	200	300
Class II, Type A:	75	260	400
Class II, Type B:	100	250	360
Class II, 100% Exhaust:	100	500	1150
Class III:	A	A	A
Laboratory Fume Hood	100	750–1000	1250–1500

A One air change of cabinet volume each 3 min for general ventilation or to accommodate heat load (whichever is greater). The cabinet must be under at least 0.5 in negative pressure, and the airflow must be adequate to provide at least 100 fpm through a glove port should a glove come off inadvertently.

    For correct sizing of the exhaust fan, the cabinet manufacturer should be consulted for the pressure drop through the cabinet with fully loaded filters. A mass airflow monitoring device should be included to warn the operator when the exhaust air quantities drop to an unsafe condition.

    e. *Certification test before use:* It is recommended that the safety cabinet be tested by a qualified individual: 1) after it has been purchased and installed but before it is used; 2) after it has been moved, relocated, or serviced; and 3) at least annually. This certification should include testing for filter integrity and efficiency, airflow velocities, integrity of the enclosure around the work area, and contaminated air plenums and relative air pressure of air plenums. Provisions are needed for measuring the flow rate and leak-checking the filters as required for certification.

2.   Secondary Barriers

Architectural and engineering features of the laboratory can form a secondary barrier to protect personnel in other areas of the building and the environment from exposure to research materials released into a laboratory room. Release of biogenic materials may result from the absence or failure of primary barriers or because of a laboratory accident occurring outside the primary barrier. The secondary barrier is not intended to reduce the risk of exposure for personnel inside the laboratory room where the release may occur.

A secondary barrier may include 1) materials and methods of construction that facilitate cleaning and prevent accumulation of contamination; 2) a pest- and vector-proof design; 3) protection of utility distribution systems from contamination; 4) treatment of liquid and air effluents to remove contaminants; and 5) air pressure gradients to maintain migration and infiltration of air from noncontaminated areas to potentially contaminated areas. The levels of containment achieved will depend on which of, and to what extent, these elements are used in the design. The National Cancer Institute has classified research facilities on the basis of contamination control features as being either a basic facility; a containment facility; or a maximum containment facility. The features of these facilities are given below.

Basic Laboratory: This laboratory provides general space in which work is done with viable agents that are not associated with disease in healthy adults. Basic laboratories include BSL1 and BSL2 facilities. These laboratories are appropriate for work with infectious agents or potentially infectious materials when the hazard levels are low and laboratory personnel can be adequately protected by standard laboratory practice. Although work is commonly conducted on the open bench, certain operations are confined to biological safety cabinets. Conventional laboratory designs are adequate. Areas known to be sources of general contamination, such as animal rooms and waste staging areas, should not be adjacent to patient care activities. Public areas and general offices to which nonlaboratory staff require frequent access should be separated from spaces that primarily support laboratory functions.

Containment Laboratory: This laboratory has special engineering features that make it possible for laboratory workers to handle hazardous materials without endangering themselves, the community, or the environment. The containment laboratory pertains to a BSL3 facility. The unique features that distinguish this laboratory from the basic laboratory are the provisions for access control and a specialized ventilation system. The containment laboratory must be an entire building or a single module or a complex of modules within a building. In all cases, the laboratory is separated by a controlled access zone from areas open to the public. Representative floor plans showing the separation of the controlled area from public areas are shown in Figure 8 on the following page.

Maximum Containment Laboratory: This laboratory has special engineering and containment features that allow safe conduct of activities involving infectious agents that are extremely hazardous to the laboratory worker or might cause serious epidemic disease. The maximum containment laboratory pertains to a BSL4 facility. Although the maximum containment laboratory is generally a separate building, it can be constructed as an isolated area within a building. The laboratory's distinguishing characteristic is that it has secondary barriers to prevent hazardous materials from escaping into the environment. Such barriers include sealed openings to the laboratory, airlocks or liquid disinfectant barriers, a clothes-change and shower room contiguous to the laboratory, a double-doored autoclave, a biowaste treatment system, a separate ventilation system, and a treatment system to decontaminate exhaust air.

E. Personal Protective Clothing and Equipment (Other than RPE)

1. Introduction

The main functions of personal protective equipment (PPE) are reduction of human exposure from infectious agents; reduction of bodily injury from mechanical or physical hazards; reduction of bodily exposure to chemicals and other toxic materials; and reduction of human particulate matter from contaminating specialenvironments. When used in a medical, pharmaceutical, or biotechnology setting, PPE should also enhance clinical technique and process hygiene. When selected and used properly, PPE promotes process quality assurance, worker task confidence, and job safety.

PPE fall into three broad classes:

- for preventing physical trauma;
- for preventing toxic chemical (solid, liquid, gas) exposures; and
- for preventing hazardous exposures to humans or their processes from agents of biological origin.

Each class can be further categorized depending on the body system it is designed to protect (e.g., eye and face protection, respiratory protection, or hearing protection), and may be further differentiated by the level of safety protection that each provides from low, to intermediate, to high performance. Other classification schemes for PPE include classification by specific occupational group (e.g., surgical or

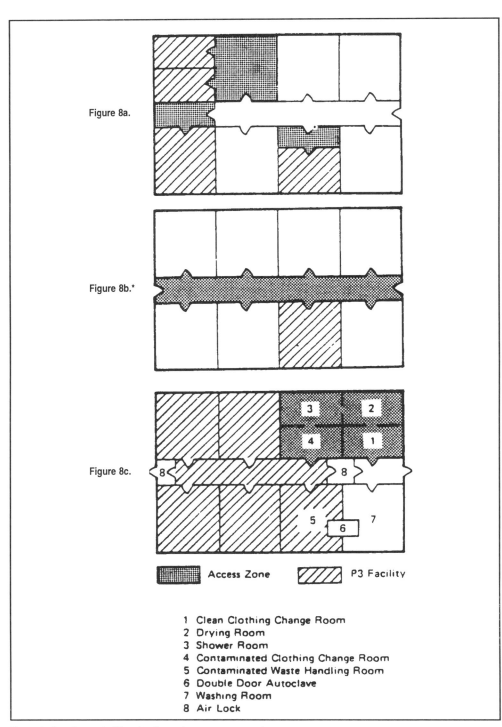

Figure 8a.

Figure 8b.*

Figure 8c.

| Access Zone | | P3 Facility |

1 Clean Clothing Change Room
2 Drying Room
3 Shower Room
4 Contaminated Clothing Change Room
5 Contaminated Waste Handling Room
6 Double Door Autoclave
7 Washing Room
8 Air Lock

Figure 8. Containment facilities showing various arrangements of space.

_____

* This approach is acceptable but undesirable unless strict access control can be ensured.

laboratory worker apparel); classification by the barrier materials used (e.g., natural materials such as cotton, leather, and natural latex, or man-made materials such as vinyl or nitrile); or classification by degree of quality assurance (e.g., nonsterile, or sterile).

2. PPE for Biohazardous Activities

Biohazardous agents include microorganisms such as bacteria and viruses; biological materials that harbor these pathogens or their toxic metabolic byproducts (such as blood and body fluids, tissues, and cell cultures); infectious animals and insects and their products; biotechnology hazards associated with the use of a living organism — or parts of an organism — to improve plants or animals, or to genetically engineer organisms for specific purposes; and particulate matter of human origin that contaminate industrial production processes.

PPE used to prevent biohazardous exposures have in common an overall purpose to prevent or control transmission of infectious or pathogenic agents. Transmission of infectious agents occurs through two major routes: direct transmission (such as direct contact) or projection via droplets directly into the mucous membranes, and indirect transmission, which includes airborne (inhalation of infectious droplet nuclei or other pathogenic particles such as allergens or endo-/exotoxins), vehicle-borne (such as in food or drink), or vector-borne (arthropods) transmission. Each mode of transmission has been associated with occupationally acquired infection. Laboratory incident reports alone from the past 100 years have documented more than 5000 cases of laboratory-acquired infections and 200 occupationally related deaths.[16]

Although most types of PPE may under certain circumstances provide for biological protection, true biological protective equipment and clothing (BPEC) have important performance characteristics that distinguish them from other forms of PPE and safety apparel. Some or all of the following key performance attributes are shared by this class of PPE:

1. BPEC are designed to interrupt infection transmission of pathogenic, pyrogenic, or allergenic exogenous biohazardous agents. Examples include those worn by health care, veterinary, and public safety workers who have direct contact with infectious tissues or body fluids.
2. BPEC are designed to prevent the contamination of special environments or products from endogenous biohazardous agents and clothing lint. Examples include PPE worn by foodservice, pharmaceutical, biotechnology, and "cleanroom" workers.
3. BPEC are designed to attenuate the effects of exposure if a biohazardous agent breaches the initial protective barrier provided by PPE. Examples include protective undergarment apparel, glove liners, or fabric treatments that reduce infection during war such as those applied to certain military uniform components.
4. BPEC are designed to preserve the human body, or to inhibit microbial growth. Examples include outer space garments, or barrier materials with surface treatments to reduce microbial growth or odor.
5. BPEC are designed to repel infectious arthropods. Examples include pesticide surface treatment of barrier materials used by outdoor sportsmen and soldiers.
6. BPEC are designed to complement other classes of PPE and barrier methods when used against extreme, unknown, or mixed hazards.

BPEC may also be used just like other classes of PPE for protection against physical and chemical hazards; however, when measured against the six performance criteria identified above, BPEC in essence perform a dual function. They provide the wearer with protection from biohazards in the external environment, and some also provide the environment protection from biohazards generated by the wearer.

3. Existing Regulations and Enforcement

In the United States there is no single comprehensive federal regulation governing PPE use for workers exposed to biohazards. However, several key standards by the U.S. Food and Drug Administration (FDA) and OSHA require that PPE be worn and stipulate certain performance requirements for equipment. Although there are numerous references to PPE in OSHA standards, few of them apply directly to protection against biohazards. The following OSHA regulations mandate important aspects of PPE usage and provide some guidance for their minimum performance in occupational settings in which biological hazards might be encountered:

21 CFR 800.20	Patient examination gloves and surgeon's gloves; sample plans and test methods for leakage defects; adulteration
29 CFR 1910.133	Eye and face protection
29 CFR 1910.134	Respiratory protection
29 CFR 1910.135	Occupational head protection
29 CFR 1910.146	Permit-required confined spaces
29 CFR 1910.156	Fire brigades
29 CFR 1910.1030	Bloodborne pathogens
29 CFR 1910.1450	Occupational exposure to hazardous chemicals in laboratories
29 CFR 1926.28	Regulations for construction
29 CFR 1926.65	Hazardous Waste Operations and Emergency Response (HAZWOPER)

These standards often refer the employer and employee to other guidelines and national consensus standards that describe appropriate barrier equipment, infection control practices, PPE performance criteria, test methods, and some selection guidance. The bloodborne pathogens standard is the most specific of the OSHA standards on protection against biohazards. Its requirements will be discussed later in this chapter.

The collective OSHA PPE standards (1910.132–137) were revised recently. The revisions were published in the *Federal Register* (6 April 1994) and took effect in October of 1994. These changes, the first in 25 years, reflect progress in industrial hygiene and occupational safety practices and in current standards by the American National Standards Institute (ANSI). OSHA expects that these revisions will most directly affect the 1.1 million work establishments in general industry and their approximately 11.7 million employees. OSHA predicts that these revisions will prevent four deaths and save 712,000 lost workdays and 65,000 non-lost workday injury cases annually. Injury and illness reduction and the prevention of worker deaths are anticipated from mandated hazards assessment activities and enhanced employee training and documentation requirements.

The new revisions expand OSHA's PPE enforcement authority into the areas of hazard assessment and worker training. In compliance with the OSHA hazard communication standard (29 CFR 1910.1200) manufacturers may also recommend specific PPE usage within spill control guidance contained on material safety data sheets. Employers would be prudent to comply with this guidance. In addition to OSHA enforcement authority, the FDA is charged with the enforcement of exam and surgical glove quality production regulations (21 CFR 800) under the requirements of section 501(c) of the Food, Drug, and Cosmetic Act of 1990 (55 CFR 51256). This regulation allows the FDA to seize noncompliant or misbranded domestic glove products and to detain imported gloves as "adulterated" products.

States and localities have laws that also apply to PPE. These laws vary from state to state, but it is not uncommon for states to control the handling, treatment, and disposal of biohazards as regulated wastes; thus, the disposal of used contaminated PPE may be subject to federal, state, and local infectious or hazardous waste disposal regulations.

4. Existing Guidelines and Standards

National guidelines and occupational safety standards pertinent to the use of PPE to control exposure to biohazards apply to the following workplaces:

- microbiological and biomedical laboratories;[17]
- research laboratories working with recombinant DNA;[1]
- "cleanroom" facilities;[18,19] and
- health care facilities, including:
  - a. hospitals and ambulatory care facilities;[10,20-26]
  - b. clinical diagnostic laboratories;[27,28]
  - c. dental facilities;[29-31]
  - d. emergency medical operations and public safety services;[32-36] and *
  - e. HIV/HBV production facilities.[10,20]

---

* The NFPA *Gloves for Structural Fire Fighting* standard (NFPA 1973)[34] includes new provisions for biological penetration resistance.

The following discussion summarizes these guidelines and provides current information about performance or test methods for barrier materials and other important considerations in each of these work settings. This discussion will not include the use, performance, and selection of chemical, physical, or respiratory protective equipment used in hazard control. Respiratory protective equipment is covered in Section F of this chapter. Employers should be aware that physical and chemical hazards often coexist with biological hazards and cannot be ignored in the PPE risk management process.

5. Microbiological and Biomedical Laboratories

The CDC guidelines for microbiological and biomedical laboratories make specific recommendations for personal protective equipment and apparel use in laboratories that are classified into four biosafety levels. BSL1 has the lowest level of biosafety risk. BSL4 has the highest level of disease and environmental hazard potential.[17] Each safety level corresponds to the "Classification of Etiologic Agents on the Basis of Hazard" contained in the NIH *Guidelines for Research Involving Recombinant DNA Molecules.*[1]

Standard microbiologic practice in both BSL1 and BSL2 laboratories requires that laboratory coats, gowns, or uniforms be worn to prevent contamination or soiling of street clothes. Special practices in a BSL2 laboratory require that laboratory coats, gowns, or uniforms be worn while in the laboratory and that before leaving the laboratory for a nonlaboratory area (e.g., cafeteria, library, administrative offices) the laboratory clothing be removed and left in the laboratory. Although it is acceptable to cover the laboratory protective clothing with clean protective clothing not used in the laboratory when leaving the laboratory for a nonlaboratory area, it should be discouraged to the extent possible since common laboratory activities involve toxic chemicals, radionuclides, and microorganisms. Wearing these garments to the cafeteria, library, or meeting place defeats the original purpose of the PPE and safety apparel and provides a mechanism for spreading contamination to other locations and persons. Standard microbiological practice also prohibits eating, drinking, smoking, applying cosmetics, and storing food in the work area. The majority of all research, diagnostic and production laboratories operate under BSL1 and BSL2 safety precautions.

Occupational safety at BSL3 relies heavily on primary and secondary containment barriers, administrative controls and facility design. Unlike organisms requiring BSL1 or BSL2 containment, BSL3 organisms can be infectious through an aerosol route of exposure and might cause serious illness and potential environmental hazard if uncontrolled. BSL3 special practices also require that laboratory clothing worn in the laboratory not be worn outside the laboratory. Front-buttoned lab coats are unsuitable.[37] Used laboratory clothing must be decontaminated before being laundered. Other forms of personal clothing such as raincoats or hats should not be stored in the laboratory work space. Entry into the lab area must be through controlled access. Only authorized persons essential to research or facility support needs are allowed access. Persons under the age of 16 may not enter a BSL3 laboratory, and animals or plants not related to the experiments are not permitted in these laboratories. General principles for handling infectious wastes and contaminated PPE such as those contained in the National Research Council's *Biosafety in the Laboratory: Prudent Practices for Handling and Disposal of Infectious Materials*[38] and the National Committee for Clinical Laboratory Standards's *Clinical Laboratory Waste Management (Approved Guidelines, 1993)*[39] are to be enforced in this work setting.

BSL4 biological agents present life-threatening potential to the worker, or they may initiate an outbreak of disease if released into the environment. BSL4 facilities are extremely sophisticated in terms of containment and decontamination design. BSL4 special practices require that street clothing be removed and stored in an outer clothes-change room. Complete sets of laboratory clothing, including undergarments, pants and shirts or jumpsuits, shoes, and gloves are provided and used by all personnel entering the facility. When leaving the laboratory and before proceeding into the shower area, personnel remove their laboratory clothing and store it in a locker or hamper in the inner change room. Soiled laboratory clothing is autoclaved before laundering. It is not uncommon for whole rooms to be designed like a Class III biological safety cabinet and for workers to walk into this area to perform tasks. The apparel worn in this situation is usually a one-piece, positive-pressure suit ventilated by a life-support system. The room is equipped with a chemical shower to disinfect the suit on exit. Access to these facilities is strictly controlled. Members of the lab staff must have specific and thorough training in handling agents and the operations of equipment and safety systems, and are provided rigorous supervision.

In its *Biosafety in Microbiological and Biomedical Laboratories* guidelines,[17] the CDC also addresses biosafety and PPE recommendations for workers in vertebrate animal research facilities. The same four-level format is used, but levels are redesignated as animal biosafety levels. Though essentially the same, three additional PPE apparel precautions are recommended for additional safety in animal laboratories. These precautions require that lab coats, gowns, or uniforms not be worn, even with over-garments, into any other facility location beginning at the level of ABSL-1; that an appropriate respiratory equipment protection program must be in place at all ABSL levels; and that at ABSL-3, only wrap-around or solid-front gowns or uniforms be worn by personnel entering level 3 facilities. The use of front-buttoned lab coats is specifically discouraged. Head and shoe covers should be available at all biosafety levels and should be worn in ABSL-3 and ABSL-4 facilities. These modifications are based on the higher levels of soiling common in animal laboratory facilities, and from the hazards of airborne allergens generated by the animals or their bedding materials. The OSHA occupational exposure to hazardous chemicals in laboratories standard (29 CFR 1910.1450) also contains similar recommendations for animal researchers to maintain higher levels of PPE precautions because of the hazards associated with incomplete suppression of aerosols. Further information related to animal research, PPE, and institutional laundering of animal worker apparel is contained in NIH's *Guide for the Care and Use of Laboratory Animals,* published in 1985.[40]

6. Recombinant DNA Research Facilities

The NIH guidelines for recombinant DNA research also require the use of protective clothing and equipment in BSL2, BSL3, and BSL4 laboratories.[1] The use of laboratory clothing is left to the discretion of the project supervisor in BSL1 laboratories. The lab director or production supervisor must make an assessment of the activities conducted and select practices, containment equipment, PPE, and facilities appropriate to the risk, regardless of the volume or concentrate of agent involved. Laboratory clothing should not be worn outside these facilities or to any nonlaboratory area within the facility. For BSL3 and BSL4 facilities, the use of area-specific colored laboratory clothing is recommended as a means for monitoring the movements of personnel, sterilization, and laundering practices, and for disposal of clothing.

All reusable clothing worn in BSL1 facilities can be discarded into a closed container and laundered in a conventional manner. Reusable clothing from a BSL2, BSL3, or BSL4 laboratory should be placed in a closed container and subsequently sterilized before laundering. Disposable clothing that is grossly contaminated should be wetted down with the appropriate disinfectant and autoclaved prior to final disposal.

7. Cleanroom Facilities

As of publication of this manual, no federal regulations require manufacturers to use cleanrooms. Manufacturers voluntarily elect to use this type of technology to increase end-product quality and establish more efficient manufacturing processes. The human body generates a "bioburden" on the manufacturing process through the constant shedding of skin cells and by the generation of moisture droplets during respiration. The resulting rate of environmental contamination increases in both forms as human activity increases. The body and street clothing also carry dust, hair, textile lint, cosmetics, perfume, and tobacco smoke particles. If uncontrolled, these forms of biological contamination can have adverse effects on manufacturing processes. To control this form of biohazard, cleanroom garments are used in the foodservice, medical implant, biotechnology, pharmaceutical, electronics, film-processing, optics, and aerospace industries.

Cleanroom apparel is used to reduce process contamination by particulate material from the human body and lint from clothing. It may also provide chemical protection from high-purity pharmaceuticals or solvents common in the semiconductor industry. There are two basic types of protective garments based on the level of quality assurance provided during manufacture: "cleaned" and "sterilized." Cleaned garments commonly are used in electronics, semiconductor, and computer industries to meet their production process needs in reducing risks from static electricity and particulates. Sterilized garments are used in medical, pharmaceutical, and biotechnology industries where assurance of sterility is important. Both woven (e.g., continuous-filament polyester yarn — not natural yarns) and nonwoven polymer fabrics are used in the construction of this apparel because of their ease of gamma irradiation sterilization. When electrical conduction is critical, there are three selection alternatives for static control in garments. These options include the use of carbon, nickel, or aluminum fibers woven into the fabric; a topical (cationic antistatic rinse) surface treatment; or biconstituant yarns that contain a conductive core fiber for static charge control. Some static dissipative or conductive gloves are manufactured to meet military performance standards for static control, such as MIL-STD–1686B and MIL-B-81705.[41,42]

Cleanroom air is classified according to federal standard 209E, *Airborne Particulate Cleanliness Classes in Cleanrooms and Clean Zones*.[43] In federal standard 209E, air cleanliness is defined by the number of airborne particles (0.5 µm and larger) per cubic foot of air. There are six common air quality classes: Class 1, 10, 100, 1,000, 10,000, and 100,000. Each class number is equal to the total acceptable number of particles per cubic foot of air. Airborne particles can be either viable or nonviable, and 209E makes no distinction on this issue. Nor does 209E define cleanliness values for objects or products (e.g., garments). Cleanroom apparel itself is manufactured in cleanrooms meeting at least Class 10 or Class 100 air quality levels.

For a Class 100,000 room, apparel includes bouffant cap or hood with full hair cover, beard cover, coveralls or zippered frock, footwear and gloves. In a Class 10,000 room, a hood replaces the cap. Class 1,000 rooms usually require full coveralls rather than the zippered frock. Class 100 requires a full head cover with open face or full-protection hoods, and a Class 10 environment demands a more complete facial coverage. The stringency of these recommendations increases with the area density of employees. An increase in the number of workers creates a corresponding increase in bioburden, and the demand for environmental regulation in terms of air filtration capacity. Flexibility in these guidelines depends on the administrative controls established by the employer for cosmetics, colognes, and perfumes, or the level of available plant technology to regulate air filtration, airflow direction, velocity and turbulence, and air volume replacement.

Cleanroom apparel manufacturers usually do not certify garments by air class ratings. Rather, employers select garments to meet specific production requirements. Garments used in pharmaceutical production facilities, however, must also comply with 21 CFR 820 specifications for food and drug handling. Selection of cleanroom apparel is based on hazards present in the work setting; normal ASTM (chemical/physical) PPE test performance standards; garment cleanliness guidelines contained in the recommended practices of the Institute of Environmental Sciences (IES) Contamination Control Division;[18] and U.S. Pharmacopeial Convention (USPC) guidelines.[19] ASTM is developing additional standard test methods, and the ANSI/ISEA 101–1993 American National Standard also provides dimension guidance for limited-use coverall size determinations.[44]

Garments used in the foodservice industries (beard covers, bouffant caps, shoe covers, aprons, gloves, etc.) are not manufactured to the same level of quality assurance as clean room apparel. Gloves must comply with FDA/USDA food processing standards for use *in contact with* food (21 CFR 177.1520) and food-coloring materials (21 CFR 175.300). Some gloves contain absorbable cornstarch as a donning lubricant. Lubricant cornstarch must comply with USPC requirements.[45] Other work wear (e.g., aprons, hairnets) do not require USDA review or approval but are subject to evaluation for acceptable performance or cleanliness standards by any USDA inspector, or by state or local public health foodservice inspectors at the point of use.

Bioprotective performance of cleanroom apparel is achieved or enhanced by:

- Fabric construction material (containment or filtration of airborne particulates larger than 0.5 microns). In general, nonwoven fabrics release less lint or particulates than woven fabrics. Multi-layered material construction provides more particle and liquid holdout than single layer construction.
- Garment design and contoured fit (minimize billowing).
- Closure design (collar, cuff, and zipper designs).
- Seam technology (serged, bound, or sealed seams).
- Antistatic finish, conductive yarn, or biconstituant yarns (reduce static electrical discharge and the tracking of particulates into clean/sterile environments).
- Cleaning, sterilization (gamma irradiation), and packaging assurance during garment manufacture.
- Concomitant use with other PPE (gloves, goggles, and face coverings).
- Surface texture. (Correct donning requires the smooth side of the nonwoven fabric to be worn on the outside. This promotes particles shedding to the floor rather than clinging to the uniform.)
- Durability to repeat cleaning (reusable garments).

8. Health Care Services

The CDC recommends using appropriate PPE as part of Universal Precautions to take when contact with blood or body fluids is anticipated.[23] The OSHA bloodborne pathogens standard defines PPE as specialized clothing or equipment worn by an employee for protection against a hazard. It further stipulates that general work clothing (such as uniforms, pants, shirts, or blouses) not intended to function as protection against a hazard is not considered to be PPE. PPE includes — but is not limited to — gloves, gowns, laboratory coats, clinic jackets, shoe covers and boots, face shields, masks, and eye protection; and equipment used in cardiopulmonary resuscitation (CPR) such as mouth pieces, resuscitation bags, and pocket masks. The standard requires that the level of protection afforded by the PPE be "appropriate" to the expected exposure. PPE is appropriate only if it does not permit blood or other potentially infectious materials to pass through to reach the employee's work clothes, street clothes, undergarments, skin, eyes, mouth, or other mucous membranes under normal conditions of use, and for the duration of use.

The performance orientation of the standard for PPE relies on the employer to select appropriate PPE. It also focuses on the issue of the effectiveness of PPE when challenged with biological hazards. Although various PPE have been used in the health care setting for many years, its actual effectiveness against microbiological penetration has been pursued most actively pursued in research since the advent of the AIDS pandemic.

Body Protection

Biomedical researchers, laboratory workers, and health care providers use combinations of components to devise an apparel system (pants, lab coats, aprons, sleeve protectors, etc.) for general body protection from daily soiling and splattering. There are disposable and reusable fabric options to meet both clinical and environmental needs. In general, reusable apparel is made from woven fabrics (e.g., cotton/polyester yarn) or nonwoven polymer fabrics. Woven fabrics are usually surface-treated to enhance liquid resistance and give them antistatic properties. Reusable nonwoven fabrics, commonly made from polyester and polypropylene, are manufactured as either spun lace, spunbond, or spunbond/meltblown/ spunbond compositions that may be reinforced with breathable or nonbreathable polymer films or coatings. Reusable apparel may be constructed of single or multilayers of similar or dissimilar fabrics and coatings. Film coating may be microporous (breathable) or nonporous (nonbreathable). Disposable apparel is most often composed of a nonwoven polymer fabric (e.g., polyester/polyolefin) constructed as a single-layer garment. The single-layer fabric, usually a spun lace, is often provided a water repellant surface treatment or antistatic finish.

The barrier efficiency of these fabrics to liquid penetration, or "strike-thru," is variable. In general, woven materials and single-layer materials provide the least amount of strike-thru protection. Reinforced or layered materials provide better strike-thru protection than single-layered garments. Garments constructed of reinforced fabrics with film or polymer coatings can achieve the highest level of strike-thru protection. Unfortunately, the comfort of these garments in terms of vapor and heat transfer is generally the converse of liquid resistance. Garments composed of nonwoven polymers reinforced with nonporous film coatings may be uncomfortable to wear for extended periods. Since strike-thru protection varies by the type of material construction used in the garment, selection must be based on the amount and frequency of liquid exposures predictable in the workplace, the overall design integrity of the garment, the liquid-resistance properties of the selected apparel material, and the overall level of integrated protection provided when multiple apparel components (such as when shoe covers, pants, lab coats, and face protection) are all worn together. To reduce exposures to the forearm from either liquid chemicals or body fluids, OSHA's bloodborne pathogens and occupational exposure to hazardous chemicals in laboratories standards recommend that long-sleeved garments be used rather than short-sleeved attire.

There are standard test procedures for determining the permeability resistance of clothing materials. Most clinical apparel manufacturers historically have used procedures to determine liquid resistance using air permeability, water repellency, and water resistance as standard protocols. Although water may be a common liquid for testing, it does not have the same physical and chemical properties as a biological fluid such as blood. Human blood possesses unique liquid properties such as a low surface tension (42–60 dynes/cm vs. 72.8 for water) that allows it to readily penetrate fabric materials. Traditional methods to evaluate liquid penetration of garments are suboptimal since they are poor models for blood penetration and they do not evaluate microbial penetration. Concern about potential exposure to microbial pathogens in body fluids has led to the development by ASTM and others of newer test methods using surrogate pathogens and fluids. Biopenetration test methods will be addressed in the glove section.

Historically, two types of general overgarments have evolved as preferred work wear in the lab setting: gowns and front-buttoned white coats. Each have benefits and drawbacks. Front-buttoned white coats look better to the worker and may project an elevated status. Coats may be easier to don and remove, especially in an emergency. If left unbuttoned they offer no protection. They may offer little protection to the legs, knees, or thighs when sitting. Open cuffs allow aerosols and spillage to enter the sleeve. Even when buttoned, some do not protect the neck area from splash. Gowns tied behind the back might be slightly harder to remove in an emergency; however, wrap-around, solid-front gowns equipped with knitted cuff designs eliminate many cross-contamination and compliance problems permitted by lab coats. Unfortunately, neither of these overgarment types is well-suited for the emergency medical service (EMS) setting where kneeling, space constraints, and other environmental hazards dictate other apparel performance. Modern one-piece jumpsuit or coverall designs are apparel systems that offer much utility and can offer integrated safety features in a variety of work settings, including those in the public safety or EMS setting.

Work with certain explosive gases, or with hot surfaces or in hot environments, may require PPE to meet additional performance characteristics. PPE may be selected that has been manufactured to meet specific flammability resistance and electrical resistivity. Where required, fabric environmental performance characteristics should comply with appropriate standards. For example, PPE fabric used in the hospital operating room where flammable anesthetizing gases are still used must comply with the federal Flammable Fabric Act (16 CFR 1610); the NFPA 99 standard for health care facilities (1993);[46] and NFPA 701, *Methods of Fire Tests for Flame-Resistant Textiles and Films* (1989).[47]

Biosafety performance of body apparel is achieved or enhanced by:

- level of quality assurance provided during manufacturing;
- material barrier effectiveness, which includes biopenetration resistance to bloodborne pathogens, liquid and hydration resistance, and general chemical resistance.
- tensile characteristics (cut, tear, and abrasion resistance);
- overall ergonomic design (fit comfort, and skin coverage area);
- overall integration of cuff, zipper, closure, and seam design technology;
- ability to reapply liquid-repellant surface finishes (woven reusables);
- durability and resistance to wear degradation if subject to reuse after institutional laundering, such as with woven cotton garments; and
- static control and flame resistance.

Face and Eye Protection

Prior to the AIDS pandemic, protective eyewear was described as the most commonly used form of worker PPE.[48] Today, glove usage in the health services sector may be a close challenger to the annual consumption of protective eyewear worn in other industrial groups. Regardless of the level of user acceptance achieved by eyewear protection products, the eyes and face of workers need to be protected from four basic hazards, including: 1) impact hazards from processes that generate projectiles; 2) splash hazards from processes that involve wet, dry, or molten materials; 3) radiation hazards from processes or natural sources that might generate electromagnetic radiation (such as laser, microwave, UV, X-rays, and gamma rays) and thermal radiation sources; and 4) eye fatigue hazards associated with visible direct light that is too bright or too dim, and glare and reflected light.

Eye and face protection is mandated by the OSHA general industry and construction standards (Parts 1910.131–133 and 1926.102, respectively). Certain levels of performance are subject to test methods established by ANSI. The ANSI Z87.1–1989 standard establishes impact and other performance standards and provides selection guidelines for eyewear and face protection devices for protection from liquid splash hazards.[49] Laser eyewear worn in the medical setting must comply with the test methods in ANSI Z87.1–1989 and ANSI Z136.1–1993,[50] ANSI Z136.2–1988,[51] and ANSI Z136.3–1988.[52] Face protection for firefighters must comply with the NFPA 1999 standard, *Protective Clothing for Emergency Medical Operations*.[33]

Biohazards challenge the protective performance of standard protective eyewear in their presentation as liquids, droplets, and aerosols. Aerosols can present a significant hazard to laboratory workers. Aerosols commonly are produced when liquids are subject to bubbling, splashing, shaking, high frequency vibration or sonic cleaning, and centrifugal forces. Hazard containment within a biosafety cabinet, ventilation, and appropriate respirators and eye protection may all be needed to control hazardous operations that involve blending, mixing, stirring, grinding, or disintegration of biological materials.

The federal bloodborne pathogens standard enhances OSHA's eye and face protection standard (29 CFR 1910.133) to include protection from exposures to mucous membranes of the eye, nose, and mouth. Health care workers and others at risk from facial splatter or splash from body fluids must protect themselves by the concomitant use of multiple protective apparel (i.e., spectacles or goggles and a clinical face mask), by a combination face mask and splatter shield, or by spectacles or goggles worn under a face shield. When full face shield devices are worn, they must be at least 6 in. in length and extend past the orbit (suborbital ridge) of the eye to prevent direct contact with the conjunctivae of the eye. Face shields are not a substitute for spectacles or goggles because they may easily allow some particles to pass around or under the shield. For this reason,spectacles or goggles should be worn under full face shields. Full face shields may be equipped with either top or bottom crowns, or both. Top crowns provide added protection against falling objects, glare, and the possibility of liquids dripping down inside the visor. Bottom crowns provide added protection to the chin and neck from flying debris and splatter. If safety spectacles are worn, they should be provided both solid side shielding and browguarding to control hazards from direct liquid splash or splatter.

The revised OSHA PPE rule on eye and face protection contained in 1910.133 mandates that protective eye and face equipment purchased after July 5, 1994, must comply with ANSI Z87.1–1989 or be demonstrated to be equally effective. Similar devices purchased before July 5, 1994, must comply with ANSI Z87.1–1968 or be equally effective.

Biosafety performance of eye and face protective devices is achieved or enhanced by:

- liquid-resistant construction;
- spectacles with solid side shields and browguards;
- goggles with indirect venting designed against liquid and airborne dust penetration;
- mask/splatter shields and goggles that extend past the orbit of the eye and that preserve peripheral vision;
- face shields with liquid-proof crown brims with overhangs that prevent fluids from dripping down inside the visor;
- ability to be easily disassembled for lens/shield replacement, cleaning, or disinfection; and
- durability and resistance to degradation if subject to reuse after cleaning, disinfection, and sterilization.

PPE for Emergency Resuscitation

The OSHA bloodborne pathogens standard defines PPE as specialized equipment worn by an employee for protection against a hazard. It further stipulates that PPE includes emergency cardiopulmonary resuscitation (CPR) equipment such as mouth pieces, resuscitation bags, and pocket masks. CPR PPE is used as an emergency temporary physical barrier between the mouth of a CPR provider and the mouth or mouth and nose of a person needing respiratory assistance. PPE may also be used by ventilator transport teams during patient transport between health care facilities. There are basically two classes of CPR equipment: the exhaled-air pulmonary resuscitators, also known as mouth-to-mouth face shields and pocket masks; and manual resuscitators, also known as bag-mask or manual pulmonary resuscitators. Pocket masks and bag-mask systems are available as either manual or powered devices. Pocket masks and bag-mask resuscitator systems cover both the nose and mouth of the victim. Mouth-to-mouth face shields cover mainly the mouth of the victim and might not always seal over the nose. Different face shield devices offer varying degrees of facial coverage. All are approved and classified by the FDA as Class II medical devices. The use of CPR and emergency cardiac care barrier devices should comply with the joint standards established by the American Heart Association and the American Red Cross,[53,54] and ASTM test methods for safety and performance (ASTM F920–85, *Minimum Performance and Safety Requirements for Resuscitators Intended for Use with Humans*).[55] Hydrophobic and bacterial filters used in face shields and bag masks have not been well-studied and their effectiveness is not clear.[56] Although CPR barrier devices are generally considered an effective barrier to prevent the transmission of most bloodborne pathogens, including HIV and HBV, there remains a theoretical risk of infection from herpes simplex and airborne diseases such as tuberculosis,[54] depending on the safety design of the device used.

Biosafety performance is achieved or enhanced in CPR protective devices by:

- liquid- and chemical-resistant construction;
- solid shielding of airway/bite block, lip, nose, mouth, and hand contact zones;
- one-way or nonrebreathing exhaust venting design;
- dome depth, conforming mask cup/cushion for face fit seal, and angular design to accommodate facial anatomical diversity and to accommodate tracheostomy, endotracheal, and nasotracheal tubes;
- transparent domes, masks, and shells to allow visualization of lip color or secretions;
- leakproof seals and leakproof cuff design;
- hydrophobic breathing filters with bacterial filter efficiency equal to or greater than 95%.
- adjustable head straps;
- capped oxygen inlet for mechanical administration of supplemental oxygen;
- mouthpiece, flexible extension tubing, and directed backflow venting to reduce rebreathing of exhaled gases;
- bag surface texturing or "tackiness" to promote grip under wet and vigorous use;
- bag tensile strength for high stroke volume and fast recycling rate;
- wide range of sizes to accommodate any adult, child, and infant;
- pressure relief pop-off valve for child and infant resuscitators;
- standardized (15 mm inside/22 mm outside) mask connector;
- ability to be assembled easily and quickly, or disassembled (if reusable) for filter, dome, cushion replacement, cleaning, or disinfection; and
- durability and resistance to degradation if subject to reuse after cleaning, disinfection, and sterilization.

Gloves

Gloves are worn as a dermal barrier to reduce worker and patient exposure to blood, body fluids, chemical liquids, and certain other physical, mechanical, radiation, and electrical hazards present in the research, health care, and laboratory settings. Generally, three types of gloves are used:

- *Surgical gloves* are sterile gloves made of latex, neoprene, or latex coated with polymer membrane or coating materials to optimize elasticity, tensile strength, ergonomic fit, and tactility. They may be provided with a dry donning lubricant. "Hypoallergenic" surgical gloves are available to reduce risks associated with latex sensitivity in the wearer or patient. These are either specially washed latex gloves or latex gloves combined with exterior layers of synthetic polymer or films materials to reduce shedding of soluble latex proteins.
- *Examination gloves* are nonsterile gloves made of latex, plasticized polyvinyl chloride, or from an expanding variety of polymerized alkene materials (e.g., polyethylene, acrylic nitrile/butadiene). They generally provide moderate fit, are usually thicker than surgical gloves, and may be obtained with or without donning lubricants. Surgical and exam gloves are regulated as Class I medical devices by the FDA.
- The third glove type is the general purpose *utility glove*. These are nonsterile gloves, usually constructed of much thicker rubber or synthetic materials such as those commonly used for housekeeping procedures. Surgical and exam gloves are intended to be used once and appropriately disposed. General purpose utility gloves may be reusable. Since utility gloves are not intended for clinical use, they are not regulated by the FDA. Certain special high performance gloves (such as lead-lined gloves common in radiology departments or cryogenic safety gloves used in clinical laboratories) can also be considered utility gloves.

Glove selection is based on a combination of objective and subjective criteria that best meet overall practice needs of the worker, the patient, and the task. The goal of glove selection is to reduce multiple chemical, physical, and biological risks to an individually determined acceptable level. The immediate objectives in the selection process are to assure to the extent possible a prolonged protective effect for the worker, control of adverse side effects to the worker or patient (nosocomial or iatrogenic infection/allergic reaction/and other injuries), and reduction in the transfer of transient microbes, endotoxins, and pyrogens to the patient, clinical and diagnostic specimens, or to the environment such as in cleanrooms.

Meeting objective selection criteria (e.g., FDA leak test certification, a unit cost objective, chemical resistance, or clinical criteria such as requirements for sterile or latex-free gloves) is often easier than meeting subjective criteria. Key subjective selection criteria include the clinical procedure; the level of barrier protection required over time; case-specific hazards presented to the clinician and to the patient; and performance characteristics such as comfort, fit, and feel. Additional subjective selection criteria include product degradation; presence or lack of anti-microbial constituents; and glove packaging considerations.

9.   Glove Performance Measurements

There are various barrier performance test methods for gloves. They include:

- visual examination (macroscopic and microscopic, including the electron microscope);
- electroconductivity;
- dye test (UV light/spectrophotometric);
- air leak tests;
- water leak tests;
- bacteriologic (*B. stearothermophilus/S. aureus*) penetration;
- viral (polio/HSV/HIV/bacteriophage ϕ-X-174) penetration; and
- radiological (iodine) leak tests.

Today there are various standard test methods, proposed test methods, and emergency test standards that specifically address barrier clothing, gloves, and microorganisms. With the exception of military specifications, all glove test methods are consensus standards.

European test standards (ENs) for protective gloves have been devised by the Committee for European Normalization (CEN)–Technical Committee 162 (CEN/TC 162). These include EN 374-1: "Protective Gloves against Chemicals and Micro-organisms (Part 1: Terminology and Performance Requirements)"; EN 374-2: "(Part 2: Determination of Resistance to Penetration)"; and EN 374-3: "(Part 3: Determination of Resistance to Permeation by Chemicals)". They are the European equivalent to the American ASTM and NFPA standards on biopenetration of gloves and other protective apparel.

For more information, contact the ASTM F-23 Technical Advisory Group liaison (Steve Mawn) at (215) 299-5521 or the NFPA staff liaison (Bruce Teele) at (617) 770-3000. The ASTM general information number is (215) 299-5585; the NFPA general information number is (617) 770-4543.

In the United States, organizations such as ASTM, NFPA, and the IES have developed similar test methods. To address concerns about holes in gloves, the ASTM D-11 committee recently revised the former ASTM water leak test methods for surgical and exam gloves (ASTM-D3577 and ASTM-3578) into a single test method — ASTM-D5151 (1990) — which increased its detection sensitivity.[57] This revised ASTM test method is essentially identical to the test method currently used by the FDA's Center for Devices and Radiological Health for leak testing and medical glove approvals. The FDA leak test method is described in 21 CFR Part 800.20.

Penetration occurs when a liquid flows through an opening — usually a micropore, molding imperfection, tear, pinprick, or faulty seam in the glove material. The initial barrier quality of gloves varies by manufacturer due to differences in material formulation (raw materials, additives, combinations) and manufacturing process (forming, stripping, drying, leaching, chlorination, lubrication, sterilization, and process control).[58] The result is the possible formation of defects in the initial barrier matrix of new gloves. The FDA leak test measures penetration, and allows for the existence of not more than a 2.5% defect rate (i.e., not more than 25 defective gloves per 1000) for sterile surgical gloves, and not more than a 4% defect rate in nonsterile exam gloves. For regulatory purposes, the FDA refers to this as the adulteration level.

Both ASTM D5151 and the FDA leak test are lab-based tests measuring manufacturing defects or holes. As such, they ensure manufacturing and marketing uniformity, and only indirectly promote enhanced occupational suitability in glove design.

Other factors that decrease fluid resistance are forces such as pulling, pushing, and twisting; the ability to withstand compression and abrasion; and the ability of a glove to resist hydration during long patient-care procedures. Clinical barrier effectiveness is measured differently in diverse work settings. The amount of fluid contact in surgery can vary depending on the anatomical site. In the public safety setting, emergency medical technicians (EMTs) face hazards from sharps and chemicals in addition to body fluid exposures. The duration of fluid-glove contact may be brief or prolonged. Duration, frequency, and nature of exposures, therefore, are key factors influencing barrier efficiency and selection.

After initial production quality assurance, any glove's performance becomes exposure event-related. Permeation is an indication of how long gloves may be worn in the presence of a neat chemical, usually expressed as breakthrough detection time and measured in minutes. Degradation is an indication of how long gloves will last under conditions of increasing hydration, and is measured as percentage of weight change. Using this type of lab data, gloves can be selected for the highest chemical resistance and degradation rating for the planned task.

Contemporary refinements in glove testing methods center on detecting blood and pathogen penetration through the glove barrier. ASTM F-23.40 committees are developing penetration test methods for determining body fluid leaks with synthetic blood, and a viral penetration test using a bacteriophage surrogate (ϕ-X-174) for the AIDS and hepatitis viruses. Test sensitivity is measurably enhanced by detecting actual pathogens rather than just air or liquid penetration. These pass/fail test methods are designated as ASTM ES (Emergency Standard) 21: *Test Method for Resistance of Protective Clothing Materials to Synthetic Blood* and ASTM ES 22: *Test Method for Resistance of Protective Clothing Materials to Penetration by Blood-Borne Pathogens Using Viral Penetration as a Test System.*[59] ES-21 incorporates a solution of synthetic blood, which has surface tension similar to that of whole blood. ES-21 is a visual screening test to see if blood will quickly soak through a barrier under pressure. It might be most useful when estimating whether a garment, such as a lab coat or surgical gown, is liquid-resistant and a potential fluid barrier. If the blood soaks through the barrier in the ES-21 test, it fails either criteria. If the blood surrogate does not visually penetrate the barrier in the ES-21 test, then the ES-22 test (which is a standardized microbial assay) is performed. This step determines whether the garment is resistant to microbial (viral) penetration.

Since it is known that a very small quantity of body fluid can carry significant (infective dose level) quantities of virus, ES-22 incorporates a virus (bacteriophage ϕ-X-174) that was selected for its size (at 27 nm, it is smaller than both HIV and HBV) and spherical morphology, environmental stability, ease of laboratory detection (detectable at 1 viral particle per mL), and the absence of pathogenic activity in man. The test is a pressure test that uses the ASTM F903 test apparatus common to chemical permeation studies. A garment passing both ES-21 and ES-22 could be considered liquid-proof and a "viral barrier," and acceptable in terms of achieving the highest level of biopenetration barrier performance. Under the performance requirements of the OSHA bloodborne pathogens standard, failure to pass the ES-21 test would indicate an unacceptable barrier for exposure protection from blood and body fluids. Passing the ES-21 test mightindicate that a garment is suitable to situations in which minor or intermittent splatter occurs. Although a passing performance in the ES-22 test demonstrates a garment that should resist higher levels of biohazardous liquid contact, the ES-21 and ES-22 tests do not evaluate the whole glove or garment. Test results only indicate *initial* biopenetration resistance. With prolonged exposure, any garment's biopenetration resistance will degrade.

At present, only a small number of glove manufacturers can produce gloves of medical thickness (approximately 0.15 mm–0.25 mm) that can pass the ES-22 biopenetration test. Exam gloves that can pass the ES-22 performance level might be considered by health care workers for a variety of applications. These include their potential use by latex-sensitive workers if they are latex-free polymer gloves; use as microbial barrier when minor skin conditions exist; when manipulating highly concentrated biological materials; or perhaps as a glove candidate for direct patient care procedures when double gloving for high risk patient care activities.

The most comprehensive performance-related garment standard for biologically protective apparel is the NFPA 1999 standard (*Protective Clothing for Emergency Medical Operations*).[33] This standard, devised for firefighters who also conduct emergency medical services, identifies performance standards for a range of ensemble components, including garments, gloves, and face protection devices. The standard includes the ASTM ES-22 test method and other test methods, including abrasion resistance, flexural fatigue, watertightness, tear resistance, heat resistance, certain chemical degradation tests, and light transmission tests. Until more sophisticated test methods are developed, a glove or garment that passes the NFPA 1999 standard can be expected to provide protection for the wearer from multiple hazards encountered in the pre-hospital environment.

10. Microbial Permeation and Penetration of Gloves

Surgical and exam gloves constructed from either vinyl or latex materials should not be regarded as completely impenetrable barriers to microorganisms. This is due to the allowable proportion of variation (defects) in the FDA acceptance quality level for surgical and exam gloves which results from the manufacturing process, and the increasing porosity of these very thin barriers over time due to the hydration effect. Hydration can cause swelling of the barrier matrix, which allows for more efficient wetting of any existing pores or defects, and this can promote increasing breakthrough properties over time. Several microbial penetration studies have demonstrated that both bacteria and virus are capable of penetrating holes in latex and vinyl gloves used in the medical setting.[60-65] However, it has yet to be demonstrated that microbial agents can permeate the molecular pore space of gloves.

The barrier efficiency of gloves can also be influenced by physical, mechanical, and chemical damage to the glove barrier. Physical damage to gloves may be caused by stretching during donning and use, electrical burns from electrocautery and laser devices, or by environmental degradation during storage. Examples of environmental degradation include the effects of heat, humidity, oxidation, ionizing radiation, ozone, and ultraviolet light from the sun or fluorescent lights. It can occur from acid and base oxidation caused by human perspiration on latex, or from exposure to certain lubricants and hand creams. Mechanical damage can occur from abrasion, laceration, and glove punctures that occur during surgical procedures and routine patient care activities involving sharp objects (bone edges, staples, scalpels, wires and needles, syringes, clamps, etc.). Chemical damage to gloves results from exposure to institutional disinfectants, solvents, liquid adhesives, and antineoplastic and other chemical and therapeutic drugs. There also are several studies that have documented the lack of awareness in glove users to a high percentage of both the permeation and penetration degradation in their gloves.[66-71] Studies of surgeons gloves[64,72,73] have demonstrated that the frequency of glove penetrations increases with both the complexity and the duration of surgery due to the effects of hydration, increasing exposure to sharps, and the cumulative effect of material fatigue caused by finger and hand flexing motion. Because sterile gloves are manufactured to higher tensile strength specifications, they may be more resistant to material fatigue than exam gloves. The rate of mechanical, chemical, and physical degradation is different between the various materials classes used to fabricate gloves, and that variation exists even between gloves of the same material class manufactured by the same company.

Most gloves fit tightly, and in the case of surgical gloves very tightly. Adverse outcomes of tight fit for long duration include friction, muscular fatigue, and occlusion and maceration of the skin. Skin irritation is not uncommon among health care workers. Gloves can exacerbate inherent susceptibility to eczema and existing skin irritation. The risk of mucocutaneous or percutaneous exposure increases as the quality of the skin barrier decreases and the level of perspiration inside the glove increases. The CDC's Universal Precautions recommend that health care providers who have exudative lesions or weeping dermatitis refrain from all direct patient care and from handling patient care equipment until the condition resolves. Some dermatologists believe that gloves should not be worn over inflamed skin unless worn for short periods and when topical corticosteroids are applied first.[74] Pregnant and immunodeficient health care providers should also strictly adhere to Universal Precautions to minimize the risk of infectious agent transmission.

Several studies have demonstrated that vinyl exam gloves leak more frequently than latex exam gloves and have less ability to reseal in the event of puncture.[63,73,75-77] In general, vinyl gloves also have less chemical and laceration resistance than latex exam gloves and offer less resistance to permeation by chemotherapeutic drugs. It is for these reasons that the Service Employees International Union has recommended to its health care employee membership that latex gloves should be used instead of vinyl whenever possible to reduce the potential for body fluid exposures.[78]

11. Double Gloving and Other Protective Measures to Improve Glove Barrier Safety

Because of increasing awareness of potential occupational risk from surgical contact with patients with infectious diseases, and the increasing likelihood of glove penetration during surgical procedures and other patient contacts, many clinicians try to improve the barrier efficiency of gloves by double and even triple gloving. Recent studies on double gloving as a means to improve barrier efficiency have shown that the double gloving of either surgical or exam gloves can help reduce, but not completely eliminate, the hazards of microbial penetration through gloves and skin exposures from glove perforation.[64,79-83] Other studies have shown that the most frequent site for hand injury from punctures of both single and double gloving are the dorsum of the hand, fingers, and thumb of the nondominant hand.[72] These data demonstrate that certain high risk surgical procedures (such as those in thoracic, orthopedic, or obstetric surgery) that involve considerable manual manipulations, numerous sharps, contact with large amounts of body fluids, or long duration, and other patient contact procedures that place increased stress on gloves will increase the rate of glove perforation. The prudent clinician in these situations may wish to take steps to reduce the risk of occupational exposure to bloodborne pathogens and reduce the potential risk of disease transmission to patients. Measures that can reduce the risk of exposures include double gloving for procedures of long duration or high risk; use of cut-resistant gloves and glove liners under the outer glove; use of blunt tip suture needles; and other techniques for hands-free passage and storage of sharp instruments. Routine inspection of gloves and regular glove changes also are recommended.

Recent experiments in novel glove construction methods have focused on strengthening high risk puncture zones in gloves or chemically inactivating viruses after a needle penetration. Unfortunately, there is as yet no commercially available glove liner or glove barrier material that will totally prevent needle puncture. Two laboratory studies have shown that gloves containingchlorhexidine glutinate or nonoxynol-9 between layers of latex can inactivate various bacteria and viruses, including HIV.[84,85] Cut-resistant gloves and glove liners are commercially available, but they are neither needle puncture-proof nor cut-proof.[86] They are cut resistant. They are useful to clinicians who do not require high levels of tactile performance but who need protection from laceration. Pathologists, orthopedic surgeons, and morticians are among the first to benefit from advances in cut-resistant fiber and fabric materials.

Gloves are imperfect barriers. Manufacturers should work toward devising gloves with fewer inherent defects and greater wear resistance. Innovative technology for more sensitive detection of holes is under development. Researchers have patented methods to create microscopic holes of known dimension. Research is ongoing to evaluate electronic methods for detecting very small holes using the inherent electrical capacitance properties of barrier materials. Detection of charged particles and electric currents through conductive liquids and gases offers promise for advancement in production quality control of both gloves and condoms. Commercial glove hole detection devices are available to the surgical community. Their practicality, detection sensitivity, and reliability are only just beginning to be scientifically assessed.

Penetration, however, only implies exposure and not necessarily disease. There is no general correlation between relative permeation/penetration rate (*in vitro*) and the relative dermal absorption rate (*in vivo*). In other words, intact human skin is an additional barrier to the transmission of microbes. This explains why, even when the glove barrier is breached, infection does not always occur. Infection depends on a combination of factors, including the dose and virulence of the infectious agent, and the host's defense mechanism.

Inappropriate glove selection, unwarranted glove decontamination and reuse, or workers otherwise misusing gloves are probably a far greater safety problem than initial manufacturing quality. No currently reported CDC HIV seroconversion data on occupational exposure to HIV reveals any case of bloodborne infection in health care workers due to an initial glove quality failure or from any other environmentally mediated mode.[87] Documented bloodborne infections have been transmitted by percutaneous or mucocutaneous exposure routes associated with either the lack of appropriate protective equipment or by needlestick or laceration through gloves. Kotilainen et al., however, suggest that possibly three cases of herpetic whitlow might have occurred from the use of vinyl gloves in 1989, prior to the FDA's imposition of higher standards for the leak testing of exam gloves.[68] It is plausible that similar undocumented cases have occurred.

Biosafety performance of gloves achieved or enhanced by:

- level of quality assurance provided during their manufacture (including overall integrity, sterility, cleaning of soluble latex proteins, and low numbers of manufacturing defects, etc.);
- material barrier effectiveness (which includes biopenetration resistance to bloodborne pathogens, liquid and hydration resistance, and chemical resistance);
- tensile characteristics (including cut, tear, and abrasion resistance);

- ergonomic design (including fit comfort and surface texture);
- cuff design and length;
- level of quality assurance provided during storage and prior to use;
- durability (if reusable gloves); and
- frequency of inspection and replacement (especially in biohazardous, mechanically stressful, or in exposures of long duration).

Shoes and Foot Protection

Sneakers, sandals, and open toe or perforated shoe construction are generally not acceptable in a lab or clinical work setting, as required by 29 CFR 1910.1450. Shoes, boots, and shoe covers can track dirt and debris into clean zones or generate unwanted dust particles during traffic movement, or during donning or doffing activities. When dust control is important, shoe covers or overboots constructed of low particulate shedding materials, antistatic finishes, and elasticized top openings and ankles or ankle straps, may reduce this hazard. In locations where explosive gas might be present, or where flammable anesthetic agents are still in use, periodic conductivity checks may be made on footwear worn in these areas to minimize the potential for static electricity. Appropriate footwear with good traction and high slip resistance is needed in locations where floors are wet or slippery. In surgical settings where copious fluid contact is predictable, the use of rubber construction knee high or hip wader-type boots might be required. All safety or special-issue shoes and boots used in controlled access areas should be identified so that they can be segregated from safety shoes used for work in other areas. In the event of overt biological or chemical contamination, the shoes should be decontaminated or sterilized by appropriate means or discarded. Information on decontamination can be found in Chapter 6 of this manual. Safety shoes (steel toe/sole) might be necessary if there are hazards from falling objects, sharps, or contact from other heavy objects. Disposable shoe covers and boots should be provided in sufficient sizes to reduce tearing when donning and be constructed of abrasion- and moisture-resistant materials. Disposable covers or boots worn in wet areas should be constructed of liquid-resistant latex, PVC, or other polymer materials. Special effort might be necessary to ensure adequate size accommodation for women or workers with especially small feet.

Biosafety performance is achieved or enhanced in protective footwear by:

- level of quality assurance provided during manufacture to reduce the generation of donning and doffing particulate contamination, and antistatic finish;
- liquid resistance (overall liquid-tight integrity);
- chemical resistance;
- tensile characteristics (including tear and abrasion resistance);
- ergonomic design, including fit comfort, and antislip surface texture of the sole; and
- design integrity and length.

12. Human Factors Affecting PPE Selection and Use

The OSHA bloodborne pathogens standard requires that PPE be provided, readily accessible, and adequate for the duration of normal use. Provision for "similar alternative" PPE devices is also a requirement to supplement PPE normally available to the exposed work force (1910.1030(d)(3)(iii)). This clause requires employers to protect workers who might be allergic to latex or who might have other physical or medical reasons that require different PPE than normal. Provision of foot protection to accommodate women's sizes or latex-free gloves are two examples. Anthropometric differences based on race, sex, physical size, physical handicaps, or medical conditions can make it difficult to accommodate certain workers. Medical assessment is an important component of any PPE risk management program. Although it is true that some worker health complications will prohibit a worker from performing duties while wearing PPE (such as certain medical conditions associated with the use of a respirator), employers are required to accommodate their work force either through engineering and administrative controls or by adequate PPE. Accommodation is important not only for biological protection and regulatory compliance but for worker PPE acceptance and compliance, and task confidence. Personal preferences should be accommodated whenever possible.

Human factors engineering methods should be used to design PPE. The design of any PPE device or garment system to accommodate the human form is equally as important as the safety provided by the barrier materials used in its construction.

13. PPE and Apparel Cost/Economic Factors

Protective equipment and safety apparel purchasing represents a considerable overhead investment for all industries. Low unit prices do not always result in lowest overall costs. Higher quality, more durable products usually perform better and last longer to offset a higher unit cost. Cost evaluations for reusable products should be based on product use-hours rather than product unit price. Total cost for the employer is measured best as a function of the product unit cost, wear life, disposal cost, savings in employee health care costs, and employee job and task confidence.

14. Integrated PPE and Apparel Risk Management Program Considerations

All PPE share certain universal safety performance criteria. PPE performance should provide for all the following:

- PPE should be appropriate for the risk involved and the conditions at the place where the hazardous exposure risk may occur;
- PPE should accommodate both the ergonomic requirements and state of health of the person who might be required to wear it;
- PPE should be capable of fitting the wearer correctly within the adjustment range for which it is designed;
- PPE should comply with any mandated performance specifications required by existing specific hazard control regulations;
- PPE should be effective to prevent or adequately control risk without increasing the level of overall risk to the wearer; and
- PPE should be durable enough to provide both the expected level of safety protection during routine use and, if expected to be reusable, to be resistant to daily cleaning and disinfection as recommended by the manufacturer.

PPE selection, use, and disposal should be part of a comprehensive employee health and safety program. Key elements of the PPE management program within an overall health and safety program include a written program based on recognized site-specific hazards and past institutional experience; a designated program responsibility to qualified person(s); PPE and apparel performance requirements in purchasing specifications; job task-oriented policy and procedures including use/reuse, decontamination, and disposal policy; written PPE and apparel purchasing, warehousing, and quality control procedures and responsibilities; PPE and apparel purchasing based on end-user input; end-user training requirements and medical qualifications; and a documented system of PPE program auditing, including any appropriate environmental surveillance, compliance monitoring, and a regular review of the total PPE program.

Any PPE program should also include continual self-assessment. A proactive PPE assessment program includes at least five steps.[88] These steps are:

1. workplace hazard evaluation (hazard assessment and exposure assessment);
2. proactive obtainment of samples of candidate PPE;
3. evaluation of candidate PPE samples using standard or field test methods against on-site hazardous agents under local environmental conditions;
4. selection of the best candidate based on regulatory requirements, performance specifications, and test results; and
5. constant monitoring of PPE performance, durability, and worker compliance in the workplace.

The initiation of a PPE program is the final step in any comprehensive risk management process. When applied to PPE, the risk management process entails the following steps:

1. formal risk assessment of the workplace;
2. application of engineering controls to eliminate or attenuate known risks;
3. institution of administrative and work practice controls, and a medical surveillance program; and
4. a proactive PPE and protective apparel safety program.

Engineering and work practice controls are the preferred methods to eliminate or minimize direct exposure with hazardous environments, processes, or hazardous agents. PPE should be considered as the last line of defense against unplanned exposure or attenuated hazards. PPE is known as the "last choice" for exposure control because:

- PPE protects only the person wearing it, whereas controlling risks at the source protects everyone in the workplace;
- theoretical maximum levels of protection are seldom achieved with PPE in actual practice, and the actual level of protection is difficult to access;
- PPE can restrict the wearer by limiting mobility, visibility, and communication, and by instituting an added weight burden;
- PPE is only effective to the extent that the wearer is correctly trained, fitted, and the PPE is properly maintained, accessible, and available in appropriate sizes; and
- there might be some hazards for which no PPE will provide an adequate control of the risk (e.g., firefighter apparel only provides *limited* protection from radiant heat and flame).

For all of these reasons, it has been the policy of OSHA and NIOSH that PPE should be used when: 1) engineering and administrative controls are not feasible; 2) when such controls are being developed or installed; 3) when emergencies occur; or 4) when control equipment breaks down.[89] There are, however, many occupational tasks in which exposure cannot be controlled through a combination of engineering and administrative controls. Indeed, there are situations when the use of PPE is the only control method available. But more often PPE should be used to complement, not supplement, other control methods such as workplace design, prudent laboratory practice and technique, personal hygiene and immunization, and the use of primary safety barriers such as biological safety cabinets.

15. Summary

Even though engineering and administrative safety controls are the first line of defense in personal protection, not all risks can be eliminated in the workplace. When it is not possible or practical to engineer out all hazards, PPE is still necessary and a valuable ally for protection against various hazards in a dynamic workplace. When procedures require PPE, it should be appropriate for the highest level of risk to which personnel or the environment will be subjected.

When biohazards are present, at least 10 risk reduction steps should be operational:

1. To the extent possible, known hazard risks should be under engineering controls.
2. Workers should be knowledgeable of these hazards and the possible routes of disease transmission.
3. Exposed workers should be properly trained in the selection, use, and disposal of each type of PPE they use.
4. Medical surveillance, record keeping, and immunization programs should be provided.
5. Workers and management must be motivated and committed to biohazard protection standards. Disciplinary action against violators should be established.
6. PPE must be available and provided in adequate types, number, and size options.
7. Reusable PPE must be maintained properly.
8. The biosafety program should be in writing, posted, and reviewed with employees.
9. Unplanned exposures and emergencies can still happen. Emergency procedures should be set up for splash, aerosol and penetration injuries, and other exposure incidents. Emergency contingency planning, training, and communication and other response equipment must be in place. Injury and near-miss accidents should be analyzed to determine PPE program correction priorities.
10. Safe work practices, handwashing, and infection control precautions must be universal.

Key guidelines and regulations that recommend the use of barrier clothing and gloves to protect against microbial exposure have been reviewed. Glove performance literature has been cited demonstrating that not all gloves are equal. Examination and surgical gloves can be perforated, resulting in microbial exposure to the wearer. Barrier perforations can be present before use, occur during normal use, or occur as a result of a cut during use. Perhaps the greatest potential hazard exists when a perforation is present, the wearer has nonintact skin, or the perforation goes unnoticed. Unnoticed perforations are common.

When feasible, bioprotective performance indicators have been provided that identify important performance and selection criteria for several key types of PPE common to biological safety. These and other guidance provided in this chapter should assist the reader in establishing better objective and subjective performance qualifiers and program management actions.

PPE and clothing selection should be justified by intended use, appropriate to the level of injury potential or disease transmission route, and be accommodating and acceptable to the wearer. Barrier efficiency should be quantified by acceptable test measurement performance against the actual hazards encountered in the workplace. After considered selection and the initiation of operational use biological protective equipment, apparel, and devices should still be part of a proactive risk management and quality assurance program.

F. Respiratory Protective Equipment

1. Introduction

The use of respiratory protective equipment (RPE) to control exposure to infectious aerosols presents some difficult challenges to industrial hygienists. The health effects of infectious aerosols are not cumulative in nature; respiratory selection criteria for particulate hazards do not necessarily apply to infectious aerosols; and the NIOSH RPE certification process was not originally designed for infectious aerosols. In May 1994, NIOSH proposed a particulate respirator certification process that included considerations for performance criteria recommended by the CDC for respiratory devices used in the health care setting for protection against *Mycobacterium tuberculosis*. At publication of this manual, NIOSH had finalized 42 CFR Part 84 certification regulations (see *Federal Register,* Vol. 60, No. 111 [9 June 1995]).

There are no NIOSH-certified respirators specifically for infectious aerosols. It is imperative that the reader have a thorough understanding of basic respiratory protection principles and good practice before selecting and using any respirator to control exposure against any hazard. Training classes sponsored by AIHA, NIOSH, and others can provide this background.

To appropriately select RPE to control infectious aerosol exposure, the reader must also understand basic concepts of microbiology and airborne infectious disease transmission. There are several excellent texts on both subjects (see the references listed in Chapter 1); however, much of what is known about occupational exposure to bioaerosols and subsequent disease transmission comes from biosafety literature documenting infectious disease transmission in standard microbiologic research laboratories (see Chapter 2). The Sulkin and Pike survey of laboratory-associated infections revealed that exposure to infectious aerosols was considered as the plausible but unconfirmed source of infection in 80% of the reported cases.[90]

The following guidelines for selecting RPE should be applied carefully, keeping the above-mentioned limitations in mind. These guidelines will discuss currently available RPE and recommendations for proper selection and use in infectious aerosol exposure situations. Ultimately, the industrial hygienist must exercise professional judgment based on what is known about RPE, the process, and the hazard.

2. The Nature of an Infectious Aerosol Hazard

Understanding the nature of an airborne hazard is one of the first steps taken before appropriate RPE can be chosen. This statement is no less true for an infectious aerosol hazard.

The infectivity of a microbiologic agent is one of the most important properties of an infectious agent. Infectivity is the ability of the agent to produce infection by invading and multiplying in a susceptible host. Dose, environmental conditions, and the route of exposure can affect the degree of infectivity of a biologic agent. Host factors such as age, race, nutritional status, predisposing conditions, and immune system status also play an important role in disease transmission; however, for purposes of health and safety, host factors must not be relied on to prevent infection, and all personnel must be viewed as susceptible to infection.

Dose

Dose is directly related to infectivity. The infective dose is the minimum number of particles or agents required to establish infection in 50% of a group of hosts of the same species. This quantity is referred to as the ID_{50}. The ID_{50} is a function of the agent, route of administration of the agent, source of the agent, and host factors. The ID_{50} is measured in test animals and provides a way to rank various infectious agents.

ID_{50} and the threshold limit value (TLV) can be linked conceptually. If the ID_{50} by inhalation in an animal model were known for the infectious agent of interest, a correction factor for species difference could be applied to assign an ID_{50} for humans. It would never be acceptable to permit an airborne concentration approaching this level.

There is limited quantitative human infectivity data via the inhalation route. Viral infectious doses are reported in units known as 50% tissue culture infectious doses ($TCID_{50}$s) which are the end point of a quantal titration of virus that infects 50% of the inoculated cell culture host. Human infectivity data exists for a 1.5 µm diameter aerosol for the following four respiratory viruses: rhinovirus type 15; coxsackievirus A type 21; adenovirus type 4; and influenza A/2/Bethesda/10–63.[91] The $TCID_{50}$s for these viruses are 0.56, 23.20, 0.42, and 2.49 respectively. In other words, human infection due to the 1.5 µm aerosol exposure resulted from approximately 0.5 to 23 times the number of virions it takes to infect cell culture.

Environmental Conditions

Airborne microorganisms must be viable to cause infection. The viability of an agent depends heavily on environmental conditions and the agent's intrinsic properties. Intrinsic properties include growth requirements (e.g., temperature, nutrients); ability to survive outside the host in a variety of vehicles (e.g., air, water, food, soil); and viability subject to environmental conditions (e.g., light, temperature, relative humidity).

Route of Infection and Disease Transmission

The ID_{50} can vary directly with the route of exposure; an agent infectious by two routes might have a different ID_{50} for each route. This discussion will be concerned only with the airborne route of infection. Transmission of infection can be broken into two broad classifications of mechanisms of transmission: direct and indirect. "Direct" transmission includes not only direct contact but also contact as spray by droplets from sneezing and coughing onto the mucous membranes of others. These droplets travel in a ballistic manner and splatter on the nasal mucosa. This route of transmission is called the "nasal route" by some microbiologists and infection control practitioners. "Indirect" transmission involves two types of particles: dusts and droplet nuclei. Dusts are defined in infectious disease literature as particles that have settled and are resuspended (e.g., from floors, bedding, or soil).

Liquid droplets containing microorganisms dispersed by coughing, sneezing, and talking vary in size from greater than 100 µm in diameter to well below 10 µm, with the mean between 10 and 20 µm.[92] Even in 90% humidity, droplets < 80 µm will evaporate before settling from a height of 6 feet. The residual droplet nuclei might contain microorganisms. Droplet nuclei 2–3 µm in size have settling velocities of 0.015–0.020 cm/sec. Aerosols of this size are capable of remaining airborne for long periods and are more likely to be inhaled and deposited in the respiratory tract. Mechanically generated aerosols in various workplace settings may result in droplet nuclei smaller or larger than those expelled by coughing, sneezing, or talking.

The preceding discussion identifies the importance of the agent's aerosol size distribution as a function of the aerosol generation process and the existing environmental conditions as well as its mechanism of infection. For example, it is known that only aerosols < 5 µm in diameter of *Legionella* spp. can infect a susceptible host; therefore, if the work process or activity being investigated generates a mist initially 20 µm in diameter, a potential airborne hazard exists given the appropriate environmental conditions, the employee's distance from the source, and other variables common in aerosol exposure assessment.

Caution is advised when evaluating a bioaerosol hazard. Most of what is known about occupational infectious disease transmission has been obtained from documented laboratory-acquired infections occurring in standard microbiologic research laboratories. In 80% of these cases, inhalation was attributed as the route of exposure. Laboratory settings represent controlled environments where physical containment devices are used, engineering controls (biological safety cabinets) are common, and specific work practices are followed by trained personnel. Even so, all infectious aerosol exposures cannot be prevented.

There is potential for infectious aerosol exposures in workplaces other than the biomedical or research laboratory. Other industries include, but are not limited to, the following: sewage treatment facilities, zoos, veterinary facilities, HIV/HBV production facilities, slaughterhouses, agricultural settings, and health care. The workplaces cited vary greatly in the level of engineering controls available. RPE might be required in these settings.

3. Surgical Masks

Surgical masks are infection control devices because they prevent the spread of infection from the wearer to potentially susceptible person(s). They are not respiratory protection devices. It is important to understand the purpose of these devices, how they are tested, and what the data mean in order to avoid confusion as to the appropriate use of surgical masks.

Surgical masks are designed to prevent patients in health care settings from acquiring an infection from the wearer's exhaled breath. They form a limited aerosol barrier between the respiratory tract of the wearer and the patient. Although they were originally designed to control the transmission of aerosolized infectious agents from the wearer to the patient, they have also been mistakenly worn to protect health care providers from tuberculosis exposure from a TB-infected patient. Surgical masks accomplish limited barrier protection for the patient by filtering large droplets containing viable microorganisms from the wearer's exhaled breath. They can be considered to be nonsealing air-purifying devices having a highly variable aerosol filtration efficiency.

The filtration efficiency of surgical masks is usually tested by one of two methods: the Greene and Vesley *in vivo* method[93] and the military specification standard MIL-M-36954C *in vitro* method.[94] The Greene and Vesley method uses the wearer's exhaled breath as the surgical mask aerosol challenge; the military specification standard uses an atomizer that generates a bacterial aerosol challenge.* The count median diameters of the Greene and Vesley and the military standard challenges are polydisperse with median diameters of about 4.5 µm and 3.0 µm, respectively.[95]

Results of both challenge test methods are reported in terms of percent bacterial filtration efficiency or %BFE. The %BFE tests reflect the number of organisms that penetrate the mask to develop colonies on culture media. Although one bacterial cell is invisible to the naked eye, it multiplies in number to form a visual colony when adequate growth conditions are met. The number of colonies that penetrate is reported in colony forming units, or CFUs. The %BFE equals the CFU penetrating the mask divided by the CFU presented to the mask × 100%. A correction for the background count must be done in the Greene and Vesley method. The aerosol used in the Greene and Vesley test consists of more than one organism, whereas the military standard contains only *Staphylococcus aureus*.

Commercially used BFE test methods have not been standardized by a regulatory agency. Results can vary due to modifications made in the test procedure but are reported by test method only, with no indications of these modifications. Because of a lack of a standardized test method, two situations can occur: 1) vastly different results for the same manufacturer's model of mask can be obtained, and 2) vastly different results can be obtained for the same surgical mask tested in different laboratories by different methods.[96] The count median diameter (CMD) and geometric standard deviation (GSD) of the aerosol challenge, the type of aerosol challenge, and the methodology used to obtain the data should be known to directly compare %BFE results and to know what aerosol size distribution the surgical mask can filter. The %BFE or % efficiency depends on the size distribution of the aerosol challenge and the procedure used.

Permission to manufacture surgical masks for use in health care settings is granted by the FDA. To obtain FDA permission, an applicant is required to submit %BFE results obtained through an independent laboratory. There are no regulations stipulating minimum %BFE. The independently produced %BFE results are not challenged unless a manufacturer's client appeals to the FDA to replicate those results. Consequently, surgical masks are manufactured with widely varying %BFE results. A comparison study of 42 commercially available surgical masks subjected to the same %BFE test procedure in the same laboratory demonstrated that surgical masks varied from 13 %BFE to 98 %BFE. A %BFE of 98 would indicate that nearly all particles described by the challenge particle size distribution are filtered out. A %BFE of 13 would indicate that not only are most particles not filtered out but the least efficiently filtered particles are the smallest ones.

The preceding information bears relevance to the issue at hand only in terms of the patient's protection (i.e., preventing infectious aerosols from penetrating the mask to the outside). Although it may be true that for most meltblown surgical mask media the filtration efficiency is independent of the mask orientation, surgical masks are not designed to seal to the face as are negative-pressure air-purifying

---

* Although still used by some in practice, this standard was canceled by the U.S. Department of Defense on April 1, 1992. It has been superseded by standards A-A 54372, A-A 54435, and A-A 51070.

respirators. Protection from aerosol exposure, biological or otherwise, depends not only on filtration efficiency of the filter media but also on leakage at the periphery of the mask. RPE can be fit-tested to ensure an adequate fit. As the aerosol challenge decreases in size, leakage becomes a more serious problem because smaller particles easily follow the gas streamline around the mask periphery into the breathing zone.

The issue of facial fit and surgical masks was examined by Tuomi.[97] The efficiency and face seal leakage characteristics of two surgical masks were measured using a test head connected to a breathing machine. Filtration and leakage were measured as a function of particle size over a particle diameter range of 0.3–10 µm. At a 9 µm particle diameter the mean number efficiency for one unsealed and sealed mask was, respectively, 98% and 52%; at 5.5 µm, it was 95% and 55%; and at 1 µm, 6% and 2%. The difference between these two situations represents the degree of face fit leakage.

To summarize, the %BFE tests of surgical masks should not be considered comparable to the parameters of filtration efficiency, fit, and protection factors reported for industrial RPE. Surgical masks do not provide respiratory protection for the wearer, and the test results reported should not be confused as indicators of respiratory protection.

4. A Discussion of RPE Selection

On Oct. 12, 1993, the CDC published in the *Federal Register* draft guidelines on the selection of RPE for use against *Mycobacterium tuberculosis*. NIOSH — in addition to supporting the standard respiratory protection practices of fit-testing the facepiece for the correct size, offering multiple size respirator facepieces to better accommodate different size faces, and user facepiece fit checks before each use to confirm correct fit adjustments — proposed filtration efficiencies equal to or greater than 95% in an unloaded state for particles 1 µm in size for flow rates up to 50 L/min. In 1989, a subcommittee of the ANSI Z88 committee on respiratory protection was charged with the task of drafting a standard for the selection and use of RPE used to control infectious aerosol exposure. At publication of this manual, a standard has been drafted but not finalized for publication. Following is a discussion of the important aspects that should be considered before selecting appropriate RPE.

Air Sampling

Potential personal exposure can be estimated from area sampling using all-glass impingers (AGIs) and various impaction samplers (see Chapter 2). Subsequent analysis then involves assays of viability reported as the number of viable organisms or CFUs per cubic meter.

Area air sampling can be performed to determine the number of particles present; however, there are three sources of error in such measurements. First, it is difficult to extrapolate personal exposures from area sampling results. Second, it often is assumed that every particle counted is or contains a biological agent, an assumption that might not be true. Third, it also is presumed that every particle counted represents a *viable* biological agent, which again might not be true. An accurate infectious particle count can be used to evaluate the level of protection required of RPE.

Size distribution sampling is advantageous in that the results may be used to evaluate the type of air-purifying RPE required, provided that the size-related efficiency of the RPE filter medium is known. It must be kept in mind, however, that the selection of RPE tested and certified according to mass penetration of a specific size aerosol is not equivalent to number penetration of the same aerosol size distribution challenge.

Filter Selection

Biological agents range in size from 0.02 to 0.25 µm for viruses, 0.3 to 0.7 µm for rickettsiae, and 0.3 to 13 µm for bacteria. Biological agents rarely exist airborne as "naked" particles; rather, they ride on other ("carrier") particles. Some examples of biological agents on carrier particles from the parent material include *Coxiella burnetii* on soil dust, hepatitis virus on stool particulate, and *Brucella abortus* on mist particulate from cell culture media.

As mentioned above, particle size sampling can be very useful in helping to make filter selection. The following three types of NIOSH/MSHA approved particulate filters are available: Dust/Mist; Dust/Fume/Mist; and HEPA. HEPA respirators with at least 99.97% efficiency against 0.3 µm particles are the only ones that meet the CDC draft guidelines for use in preventing transmission of TB in health care facilities. NIOSH had also proposed a new method of testing particulate respirators for three different levels of filter efficiency (Types A, B, C) and for solid only (S) or both liquid and solid (L&S) particulates. Type A was proposed as the highest level of filter efficiency; however, all three types would meet the CDC draft guidelines for TB.

It is important to note here that respirator testing and certification testing procedures measure aerosol penetration in terms of mass as opposed to the number of particles. It is number penetration that is the critical parameter in determining the filter's efficiency against an infectious aerosol.

Fit

Proper fit is another important parameter for tight-fitting (i.e., half or full facepiece) air-purifying RPE. Poor fit can reduce the protection furnished by all tight-fitting respirators; therefore, it is very important to include either qualitative or quantitative fit-testing in the respiratory protection program if tight-fitting RPE is used. Note that fit-testing does not determine protection received but rather assesses respirator fit only. Fit-test methods have been described elsewhere.[98]

Items such as temple bars of glasses, skull caps, surgical masks worn under a respirator, or facial features such as facial hair or missing dentures, will add to the leakage experienced in the face-to-facepiece seal of tight-fitting RPE.

Protection Factors

Based on workplace protection factor studies and quantitative fit-testing results, protection factors have been assigned to the various classes of respirators. The protection factor for a respirator is defined as the concentration of airborne contaminant outside the respirator divided by the concentration of the contaminant inside the respirator. An assigned protection factor (APF) is the minimum expected workplace level of respiratory protection that would be provided by a properly functioning respirator or class of respirators to a large percentage of properly fitted and trained users.[99] The maximum use concentration for a respirator generally is determined by multiplying a contaminant's exposure limit by the protection factor assigned to the respirator. As mentioned above, exposure limits have not been established for infectious aerosols, but respirators can be used to achieve reductions in exposure levels. Although it is impossible to ensure that proper use of the respirator will eliminate infection in all workers, the risk of infection can be reduced.

Protection factors can be used to rate respirators. It may be difficult to say that the APF used for chemical exposure will be the same APF achieved when exposed to infectious aerosols. The APF is a dimensionless number, but there could be differences between APFs determined by mass methods as opposed to those determined by count methods. RPE with an APF of 50, however, is generally more protective than RPE with an APF of 10. NIOSH's *Guide to Industrial Respiratory Protection* (DHHS Publication No. 87–116)[100] and ANSI's American National Standard for Respiratory Protection (Z88.2–1992)[101] are two sources of generally accepted guidance on APF values for RPE. These numbers can be used to guide the health and safety professional in selecting the appropriate RPE.

Data in the literature assess the performance of RPE with respect to the critical parameter of bioaerosol particle number in actual use conditions.[102] The aerosol challenge was endospores of *Bacillus subtilis*. The study used four types of samplers with varying sampling efficiency to evaluate the protection factors of various respirators tested. The samplers included a mouth collector, nose collector, oronasal sampler, and oronasal inhalation sampler. The investigatorsreported that a penetration of 0.002% could be detected with a challenge of 1×10^5 spores per liter of air (i.e., 200 spores per liter of air). The aerosol challenge had a mass median diameter of particles of 2.1 μm with 95% of the particles between 1 and 5 μm. Although 200 spores of *Bacillus subtilis* with this size distribution might not be hazardous, 200 particles containing another organism could present a potentially infectious hazard.

Respirator Decontamination

RPE should be cleaned and disinfected regularly. Disinfection is required when RPE is used by more than one person. Disinfectants such as quaternary compounds, iodophors, and hypochlorite solutions used for this purpose generally are effective against wearer-generated contaminants. If, however, the environment contains a known biological agent(s) that might have contaminated the exterior of the respirator, then the decontamination procedure should be specific for that agent. No one disinfectant can be used for all agents. Refer to Chapter 6 of this manual for additional information on decontamination. It is important to ensure that the disinfectant will not damage the nondisposable respirator. Another option is to use disposable RPE, if appropriate, and dispose of it after use in accordance with accepted procedures. It also may be necessary to decontaminate the respirator prior to disposal.

Special consideration should also be given to proper procedures for removing contaminated clothing used in conjunction with RPE. For example, if doffing an air suit, it should first be sprayed with the appropriate disinfectant and warm water, worn wet for the appropriate contact time, and then removed. This procedure is followed to avoid exposure to the agent from the exterior of the suit that might be resuspended during suit removal.

Respiratory Protection Program

To ensure the proper use of respirators, a respiratory protection program must be implemented. The program should include standard operating procedures, hazard analysis, RPE selection criteria, training, fit-testing, maintenance including decontamination, program evaluation, and medical evaluation of respirator wearers.[98] The purpose of medical evaluation is to determine whether the user is physically capable of wearing the RPE while performing the job.

A medical surveillance program may also be used to determine whether any employees at risk of exposure — regardless of respirator use — has become infected. Such medical surveillance may include initial preplacement and periodic serological testing. This may also be used to evaluate the effectiveness of the respirators selected and the overall functioning of the program. It is possible that other tasks or job duties not requiring the use of respirators could be the source of infection for an individual.

5.   Suggestions for Selection of Appropriate RPE

Selecting the proper RPE to control infectious aerosol exposure is a difficult challenge given our present ability to evaluate the hazard. The development of a specific strategy will be case-specific and depends primarily on the infectious agent involved and the processes by which an infectious aerosol can be formed.

   a. ***Evaluate the Nature of the Hazard and Process:*** The potential for the presence of infectious aerosol must be determined. The parent material from which the aerosol is generated should be evaluated for infectious agents. The process should be evaluated for its ability to generate aerosol. Machines or instruments such as drills, saws, cutters, and compressed air jets are potential aerosol generators.
   b. ***Evaluate the Likelihood of Transmission:*** Much of the preceding discussion has centered around air-purifying RPE, although clearly other RPE having higher APFs for traditional particulate hazards may be used. This decision depends on a complete assessment of the hazard and process.

Review the literature for any evidence of transmission by inhalation. Determine whether the infectious dose by inhalation is known. Caution dictates, however, that all pathogens should be considered as infectious by the respiratory route. The employees' exposures should be assessed, considering proximity to operation and duration of exposure. If possible, air sampling should be performed to identify the agent(s), determine the number of infectious particles, and characterize the aerosol size distribution.

6.   Summary

This section has attempted to introduce general concepts of infectious aerosol exposure such as infectivity and host factors. There was a general discussion of infectious aerosol hazards to demonstrate how the differences between these hazards and other aerosol hazards hamper our ability to select RPE using a traditional industrial hygiene approach. Although there are many occupations in which infectious aerosol hazards exist, the potential for exposure among health care workers is perhaps the most readily recognized. Because of the mistaken perception among health care workers that surgical masks function as RPE as well as infection control devices, a discussion of surgical masks was included. The major issues of RPE selection against infectious aerosols were discussed, followed by suggestions on how RPE might be chosen.

References

1. **U.S. Department of Health and Human Services, National Institutes of Health:** *Guidelines for Research Involving Recombinant DNA Molecules (NIH Guidelines).* Bethesda, Md.: National Institutes of Health, 1994. [Published in *Federal Register* 5 July 1994 (59 FR 34496), with Amendments 28 July 1994 (59 FR 40170) and 27 April 1995 (60 FR 20726).]

2. **Organisation for Economic Co-operation and Development:** *Safety Considerations for Biotechnology.* Paris: Organisation for Economic Co-operation and Development, 1992.

3. **Goldman, R.H.:** Medical Surveillance in the Biotechnology Industry. *Occup. Med. State Art Rev. 6(2):*209-226 (1991).

4. **Ashford, N.A., C.J. Spadafor, D.B. Hattis, and C.C. Caldart:** *Monitoring the Worker for Exposure and Disease: Scientific, Legal, and Ethical Considerations in the Use of Biomarkers.* Baltimore, Md.: Johns Hopkins University Press, 1990.

5. **Halperin, W.E., J. Ratcliffe, T.M. Frazier, L. Wilson, S.P. Becker, and P.A. Schulte:** Medical Screening in the Workplace: Proposed Principles. *J. Occup. Med. 28(8):*547-552 (1986).

6. **Landrigan, P.J., M.L. Cohen, W. Dowdle, L.J. Elliot, and W.E. Halperin:** Medical Surveillance of Biotechnology Workers: Report of the CDC/NIOSH Ad Hoc Working Group on Medical Surveillance for Industrial Applications of Biotechnology. *Recomb. DNA Tech. Bul. 5(3):*133-138 (1982).

7. **Hawkins, N.C., S.K. Norwood, and J.C. Rock:** *A Strategy for Occupational Exposure Assessment.* Akron, Ohio: American Industrial Hygiene Association, 1991.

8. **Sullivan, J.F.:** Employee Health Surveillance Programs. In *Laboratory Safety: Principles and Practices* (edited by B.M. Miller, D.H.M. Groschel, J.H. Richardson, D. Vesley, J.R. Songer, R.D. Housewright, and W.E. Barkley). Washington, D.C.: American Society for Microbiology, 1986. pp. 20-26.

9. **American Conference of Governmental Industrial Hygienists:** *1993-1994 Threshold Limit Values for Chemical Substances and Physical Agents and Biological Exposure Indices.* Cincinnati, Ohio: American Conference of Governmental Industrial Hygienists, 1993. p. 32.

10. "Occupational Exposure to Bloodborne Pathogens," *Code of Federal Regulations,* Title 29, Part 1910.1030. 1992.

11. **Health and Safety Executive, Advisory Committee on Genetic Manipulation:** Guidelines for the Health Surveillance of Those Involved in Genetic Manipulation at Laboratory and Large Scale. *Guidance Note ACGM 4* (1982).

12. **Young, G.S.:** The Requirements and Pitfalls of Laboratory Worker Medical Surveillance. In *Health and Safety for Toxicity Testing; Symposium on Chemistry and Safety for Toxicity Testing of Environmental Chemical* (edited by D.B. Walters and C.W. Jameson). Stoneham, Mass.: Butterworth Publishers, 1984. pp. 159-181.

13. **Rake, B.W.:** Influence of Crossdrafts on the Performance of a Biological Safety Cabinet. *Appl. Env. Microbiol. 36(2):*278-283 (1978).

14. **Stuart, D.G., T.J. Greenier, R.A. Rumery, and J.M. Eagleson, Jr.:** Survey, Use and Performance of Biological Safety Cabinets. *Am. Ind. Hyg. Assoc. J. 43(4):*265-270 (1982).

15. **Stuart, D.G., M.S. First, R.L. Jones, Jr., and J.M. Eagleson, Jr.:** Comparison of Chemical Vapor Handling by Three Types of Class II Biological Safety Cabinets. *Part. Microbial. Cont.* (March/April 1983).

16. **Collins, C.H.:** *Laboratory-Acquired Infections,* 3rd Ed. London: Butterworth-Heinemann Ltd. Publisher, 1993. p. 1.

17. **U.S. Department of Health and Human Services:** *Biosafety in Microbiological and Biomedical Laboratories* (DHHS Pub. No. (CDC) 93-8395). 1993.

18. **Institute of Environmental Sciences:** *IES Handbook of Recommended Practices — Contamination Control Division.* Mount Prospect, Ill.: Institute of Environmental Sciences, 1993.

19. **U.S. Pharmacopeial Convention:** Microbial Evaluation and Classification of Clean Rooms and Clean Zones. *Pharmacopeial Forum 18(5):*4042-4054 (1992).

20. **Centers for Disease Control:** Recommendations for Prevention of HIV Transmission in Healthcare Settings. *MMWR 36 (Suppl. No. 2S):*35-185 (1987).

21. **Garner, J.S., and B.P. Simmons:** *CDC Guidelines for Isolation Precautions in Hospitals* (DHHS Publication No. (CDC) 83-8314). Atlanta, Ga.: Centers for Disease Control, 1983.

22. **Garner, J.S., and M.S. Favero:** *Guidelines for Handwashing and Hospital Environmental Control* (DHHS Publication No. (CDC) 99-1117). Atlanta, Ga.: Centers for Disease Control, 1985.

23. **Centers for Disease Control:** Update: Universal Precautions for Prevention of Transmission of Human Immunodeficiency Virus, Hepatitis B Virus, and Other Bloodborne Pathogens in Health-Care Settings. *MMWR 37:*377-382;387-388 (1988).

24. **Centers for Disease Control:** Guidelines for Prevention of Transmission of Human Immunodeficiency Virus and Hepatitis B Virus to Health-Care and Public Safety Workers. *MMWR 38 (Suppl. No. S-6):*1-37 (1989).

25. **Centers for Disease Control:** Guidelines for Preventing Transmission of Tuberculosis in Health-Care Settings, with Special Focus on HIV-Related Issues. *MMWR 39(RR-17):* (1990).

26. **Centers for Disease Control:** Guidelines for Prevention of Transmission of Human Immunodeficiency Virus and Hepatitis B Virus During Exposure-Prone Procedures. *MMWR 40(RR-8):*(1991).

27. **National Committee for Clinical Laboratory Standards:** *Protection of Laboratory Workers from Infectious Disease Transmitted by Blood, Body Fluids, and Tissue — Second Edition* (Proposed Guidelines, 1991 [NCCLS Document M29-T2, Vol. 11, No. 14. 1991]).

28. **National Committee for Clinical Laboratory Standards:** *Protection of Laboratory Workers from Instrument Biohazards* (Proposed Guideline, 1991 [NCCLS Document I17-P, Vol. 11, No. 15, 1991.])

29. **Centers for Disease Control:** Recommended Infection Control Practices for Dentistry, 1993. *MMWR 41(RR-8):*(1993).

30. **Cottone, J.A., and J.A. Molinari:** State-of-the-Art Infection Control in Dentistry. *J. Am. Dent. Assoc. 122:*33-41 (1991).

31. **U.S. Department of Health and Human Services:** *Infection Control File: Practical Infection Control in the Dental Office — A Handbook for the Dental Team.* Atlanta, Ga./Rockville, Md.: CDC/FDA, 1993.

32. **National Fire Protection Association:** *Fire Department Infection Control Program* (ANSI/NFPA 1581–1991) Quincy, Mass.: National Fire Protection Association, 1991.

33. **National Fire Protection Association:** *Protective Clothing for Emergency Medical Operations* (ANSI/NFPA 1999–1992). Quincy, Mass.: National Fire Protection Association, 1992.

34. **National Fire Protection Association:** *Gloves for Structural Fire Fighting* (ANSI/NFPA 1973–1993). Quincy, Mass.: National Fire Protection Association.

35. **OnGUARD:** *Silent War: Infection Control for Emergency Responders.* Fort Collins, Colo.: OnGUARD Inc., 1993.

36. **Zimmerman, L., M. Neuman, and D. Jurewicz:** *Infection Control for Prehospital Care Providers.* 2nd Ed. Grand Rapids, Mich.: Mercy Ambulance Service, 1993.

37. **Liberman, D.F., and R. Fink:** "Containment Considerations for the Biotechnology Industry." In *Occupational Medicine State of the Art Reviews: The Biotechnology Industry* (edited by A.M. Ducatman and D. Liberman). Philadelphia: Hanley and Belfus, Inc., 1991. Vol. 6, Issue 2, pp. 271-283.

38. **National Research Council:** *Biosafety in the Laboratory: Prudent Practices for Handling and Disposal of Infectious Materials.* Washington, D.C.: National Academy Press, 1989.

39. **National Committee for Clinical Laboratory Standards:** *Clinical Laboratory Waste Management* (Approved Guidelines, 1993) [NCCLS Document GP5-A, Vol. 13, No. 22, 1993]).

40. **U.S. Department of Health and Human Services, National Institutes of Health:** *Guide for the Care and Use of Laboratory Animals* (NIH Publication No. 85-23, Rev. 1985). Bethesda, Md.: National Institutes of Health, 1985.

41. **U.S. Department of Defense:** *Electrostatic Discharge Control Program for Protection for Electrical and Electronic Parts* (MIL-STD-1686B). Washington, D.C.: U.S. Department of Defense, 1992.

42. **U.S. Department of Defense:** *Barrier Materials, Flexible, Electrostatic Protective, Heat Sealable* (MIL-B-81705). Washington, D.C.: U.S. Department of Defense, 1989.

43. **General Services Administration:** *Airborne Particulate Cleanliness Classes in Cleanrooms and Clean Zones* (FS209E). Washington, D.C.: General Services Administration, 1992.

44. **Industrial Safety Equipment Association:** *Limited-Use and Disposable Coveralls — Size and Labeling Requirements* (ANSI/ISEA 101–1993). New York: American National Standards Institute, 1993.

45. **U.S. Pharmacopeial Convention:** *United States Pharmacopeia XXII.* Rockville, Md.: U.S. Pharmacopeial Convention, 1990.

46. **National Fire Protection Association:** *Health Care Facilities* (ANSI/NFPA 99–1993). Quincy, Mass.: National Fire Protection Association, 1993.

47. **National Fire Protection Association:** *Methods of Fire Tests for Flame-Resistant Textiles and Films* (NFPA 701). Quincy, Mass.: National Fire Protection Association, 1989.

48. **U.S. Congress, Office of Technology Assessment:** *Preventing Illness and Injury in the Workplace* (OTA-H-256). Washington D.C.: Office of Technology Assessment, 1985. p. 162.

49. **American National Standards Institute:** *Practice for Occupational and Educational Eye and Face Protection* (ANSI Z87.1–1989). New York: American National Standards Institute, 1989.

50. **American National Standards Institute:** *Safe Use of Lasers* (ANSI Z136.1–1993). New York: American National Standards Institute, 1993.

51. **American National Standards Institute:** *Safe Use of Lasers Optical Fiber Communications Systems Utilizing Laser Diode and LED Sources* (ANSI Z136.2–1988). New York: American National Standards Institute, 1988.

52. **American National Standards Institute:** *Safe Use of Lasers in Health Care Facilities* (ANSI Z136.3–1988). New York: American National Standards Institute, 1988.

53. **American Heart Association, Emergency Cardiac Care Committee:** Standards and Guidelines for Cardiopulmonary Resuscitation and Emergency Cardiac Care. *JAMA 255:*2905-3044 (1986).

54. **American Heart Association, Emergency Cardiac Care Committee:** Risk of Infection During CPR Training and Rescue: Supplemental Guidelines. *JAMA 262:*2714-2715 (1989).

55. **ASTM:** *Minimum Performance and Safety Requirements for Resuscitators Intended for Use with Humans* (ASTM F920–85). Philadelphia: ASTM, 1985.

56. **ECRI:** Exhaled-Air Pulmonary Resuscitators, and Disposable Manual Pulmonary Resuscitators. *Health Devices 18(10):*333-352 (1989).

57. **ASTM:** *Test Methods for Detection of Holes in Medical Gloves* (ASTM-D5151). Philadelphia: ASTM, 1990.

58. **Mellstrom, G.A., and A.S. Boman:** "Gloves: Types, Materials, and Manufacturing." In *Protective Gloves for Occupational Use* (edited by G.A. Mellstrom, J.E. Wahlber, and H.I. Maibach). Boca Raton, Fla.: CRC Press, 1994. pp. 21-35.

59. **ASTM:** *Atmospheric Analysis of Occupational Health and Safety Protective Clothing* (Annual Book of ASTM Standards, Vol. 11.03). Philadelphia: ASTM, 1993.

60. **Gerhardt, G.G.:** Results of Microbiological Investigations on the Permeability of Procedure and Surgical Gloves. *Zbl. Hyg.188:*336-342 (1989).

61. **Kotilainen, H.R., J.P. Brinker, J.L. Avato, and N.M. Gant:** Latex and Vinyl Examination Gloves — Quality Control Procedures and Implications for Health Care Workers. *Arch. Intern. Med. 149:*2749-2753 (1989).

62. **Dalgleish, A.G., and M. Malkovsky:** Surgical Gloves as a Mechanical Barrier against Human Immunodeficiency Viruses. *Brit. J. Surg. 75:*171-172 (1988).

63. **Korniewicz, D.M., B.E. Laughon, W.H. Cyr, C.D. Lytle, and E. Larson:** Leakage of Virus Through Used Vinyl and Latex Examination Gloves. *J. Clin. Microbiol. 28(4):*787-788 (1990).

64. **McLeod, G.G.:** Needlestick Injuries at Operations for Trauma — Are Surgical Gloves an Effective Barrier? *J. Bone and Joint Surgery 71-B(3):*489-491 (1989).

65. **Brough, S.J., T.M. Hunt, and W.W. Barrie:** Surgical Glove Perforations. *Brit. J. Surg. 75(10):*317 (1988).

66. **Dodds, R.D.A., P.J. Guy, A.M. Peacock, S.R. Duffy, S.G.E. Barker, and M.H. Thomas:** Surgical Glove Perforation. *Brit. J. Surg. 75(10):*966-968 (1988).

67. **Marin, J., A.Z. Dragas, and B. Mavsar:** Virus Permeation of Protective Gloves Used in Medical Practice. *Zbl. Hyg. 191:*516 (1991).

68. **Kotilainen, H.R., J.L. Avato, and N.M. Gant:** Latex and Vinyl Nonsterile Examination Gloves — Status Report on Laboratory Evaluation of Defects by Physical and Biological Methods. *Appl. Environ. Microbiol. 56:*1627 (1990).

69. **Palmer, J.D., and J.W.S. Rickett:** The Mechanisms and Risks of Surgical Glove Perforation. *J. Hosp. Infect. 22:*279 (1992).

70. **Wright, J.G., A.J. McGreer, D. Chyatte, and D.F. Ransohoff:** Mechanisms of Glove Tears and Sharp Injuries Among Surgical Personnel. *JAMA 266:*1668 (1991).

71. **Shanson, D.:** The Risks of Transmission of the HTLV-III and Hepatitis B Virus in the Hospital. *Infect. Control 7:*128 (1986).

72. **Cole, R.P, and D.T. Gault:** Glove Perforation During Plastic Surgery. *Brit. J. Plast. Surg. 42(4):*481 (1989).

73. **Colligan, S.A., and S.A. Horstman:** Permeation of Cancer Chemotherapeutic Drugs Through Glove Materials Under Static and Flexed Conditions. *Appl. Occup. Environ. Hyg. 5:*848 (1990).

74. **Taylor, J.S.:** "Other Reactions from Gloves." In *Protective Gloves for Occupational Use* (edited by G.A. Mellstrom , J.E. Wahlber, and H.I. Maibach). Boca Raton, Fla.: CRC Press, 1994. p. 256.

75. **Korniewicz, D.M., M. Kirwin, K. Cresci, S. Tiam Sing, J. Tay Eng Choo, M. Wool, and E. Larson:** Barrier Protection with Examination Gloves: Double versus Single. *Am. J. Infection Control 22(1):*12 (1994).

76. **Olsen, R.J., P. Lynch, M.B. Coyle, J. Cummings, T. Bokete, and W.E. Stamm:** Examination Gloves as Barriers to Hand Contamination in Clinical Practice. *JAMA 270(3):*350-353 (1993).

77. **Klein, R.C., E. Party, and E.L. Gershey:** Virus Penetration of Examination Gloves. *BioTechniques 9(2):*196-199 (1990).

78. **Service Employees International Union:** *HIV/AIDS and the Health-Care Worker,* 6th Ed. [Brochure.] Washington, D.C.: Service Employees International Union, 1991. p. 8.

79. **Matta, H., A.M. Thompson, and J.B. Rainey:** Does Wearing Two Pairs of Gloves Protect Operating Theater Staff from Skin Contamination? *Brit. Med. J. 297:*597 (1988).

80. **Carl, M., D.P. Francis, D.L. Blakey, and J.E. Maynard:** Interruption of Hepatitis B Transmission by Modification of a Gynecologist's Surgical Technique. *Lancet 1:*731 (1982).

81. **Quebbeman, H., G.L. Telford, K. Wadsworth, S. Hubbard, and M.S. Goodman:** Double Gloving: Protecting Surgeons from Blood Contamination in the Operating Room. *Arch. Surg. 127:*213-217 (1992).

82. **Gani, J.S., P.F. Anseline, and R.L. Bissett:** Efficacy of Double versus Single Gloving in Protecting the Operating Team. *Aust. N.Z. J. Surg 60:*171-175 (1990).

83. **Hussain, S.A., A.B.A. Latif, and A. Choudhary, A.:** Risk to Surgeons — A Survey of Accidental Injuries During Operations. *Brit. J. Surg. 75:*314 (1988).

84. **Modak, S., L. Sampath, H.S.S. Miller, and J. Millman:** Rapid Inactivation of Infectious Pathogens by Chlorhexidine-coated Gloves. *Infect. Control Hosp. Epidemiol. 13:*463 (1992).

85. **Johnson, G.K., T. Nolan, H.C. Wuh, and W.S. Robinson:** Efficacy of Glove Combinations in Reducing Cell Culture Infection after Glove Puncture with Needles Contaminated with Human Immunodeficiency Virus Type 1. *Infect. Control Hosp. Epidemiol. 12:*435 (1991)

86. **Fisher, A.A.:** Protective Value of Surgical Gloves including the "Cut Resistant Variety." *Cutis 49:*310-312 (May 1992).

87. **Hansen, D.J. (ed.):** *The Work Environment — Healthcare, Laboratories, and Biosafety, Volume Two.* Boca Raton, Fla.: CRC Press, 1993. p. 74.

88. **U.S. Department of Health and Human Services:** *A Guide for Evaluation of the Performance of Chemical Protective Clothing* (NIOSH Publication 90-109). Washington, D.C.: U.S. Government Printing Office, 1990.

89. **U.S. Department of Health and Human Services:** *Guidelines for Protecting the Safety and Health of Health Care Workers* (NIOSH Publication No. 88-119). Washington, D.C.: U.S. Government Printing Office, 1988. Sec. 2, p. 13.

90. **Pike, R.M.:** Laboratory-Associated Infections: Summary and Analysis of 3,921 cases. *Health Lab. Sci. 13:*105-114 (1976).

91. **Knight, V.:** Viruses as Agents of Airborne Contagion. In *Annals of New York Academy of Sciences.* New York: New York Academy of Sciences, 1980. pp. 147-156.

92. **Hatch, T.F., and P. Gross:** *Pulmonary Deposition and Retention of Inhaled Aerosols.* New York: Academic Press, 1964. pp. 137-139.

93. **Greene, V.W., and D. Vesley:** Method for Evaluating Effectiveness of Surgical Masks. *J. of Bacteriol. 83:*663-667 (1962).

94. **U.S. Department of Defense:** *Military Specification: Mask, Surgical, Disposable* (MIL-M-36954C). Washington, D.C.: U.S. Department of Defense, 1975. pp. 1-24.

95. **Friedrichs, W.H.:** Measuring Face Mask Performance: A Real Test. *J. Environ. Sciences:*33-39 (1989).

96. **3M Company:** *Technical Update 2: Laser Plume Issues.* [Product Bulletin.] St. Paul, Minn.: 3M Company, 1989.

97. **Tuomi, T.:** Face Seal Leakage of Half Masks and Surgical Masks. *Am. Ind. Hyg. Assoc. J. 46(6):*308-312 (1985).

98. **Colton, C.E., L.R. Birkner, and L.M. Brosseau (eds):** *Respiratory Protection: A Manual and Guideline,* 2nd Rev. Ed. Akron, Ohio: American Industrial Hygiene Association, 1991.

99. **Guy, H.P.:** Respirator Performance Terminology. [Letter to the Editor.] *Am. Ind. Hyg. Assoc. J. 46(6):*B22-B24 (1985).

100. **National Institute for Occupational Safety and Health:** *Guide to Industrial Respiratory Protection* (DHHS Publication No. 87-116). Cincinnati, Ohio: National Institute for Occupational Safety and Health, 1987.

101. **American National Standards Institute:** *Respiratory Protection* (ANSI Z88.2–1992). New York: American National Standards Institute, 1992.

102. **Guyton, M.C.E., H.M. Decker, and W.A. Burgess:** Techniques for Evaluating Biological Penetration of Respiratory Masks on Human Subjects. *Am. Ind. Hyg. Assoc. J. 28:*462-467 (1967).

6. Decontamination and Disposal of Biohazardous Materials

A. Decontamination and Disinfection

Decontamination can be defined as the reduction of microorganisms to an acceptable level. The process of decontamination can be achieved by either disinfection or sterilization. These terms are often used synonymously, but a clear separation of the two should be made. Disinfection is the reduction of the number of infectious organisms below the level necessary to cause infection. Inherent in this definition is the fact that some organisms might survive the activity of the disinfectant, particularly the bacterial spore-forming organisms. Sterilization, on the other hand, is defined as the complete killing of all organisms. This is an important distinction when one is faced with the decision of decontamination of materials or facilities.

It is generally accepted that materials contaminated with infectious agents must be decontaminated prior to reuse or disposal. The goal of decontamination is not only the protection of personnel and the environment from exposure to biological agents, but also the prevention of contamination of experimental materials and products by microorganisms that are ubiquitous in nature. The level of decontamination necessary depends on a number of factors, and it is important that some type of risk analysis be done to determine the most effective and reasonable method to reach the desired result. The user must decide whether the contamination is a risk to the personnel using the materials, to the materials themselves (i.e., medical devices, research materials), or to the environment (i.e., release to the air); what that risk is (based on the type of organisms present and the potential for exposure); and which method of decontamination is the most effective for that situation with the least deleterious impact on personnel, product, and the environment.

Decontamination processes, whether they involve disinfection or physical sterilization (i.e., heat or radiation), are processes that destroy tissue. Personnel exposure to the chemical and physical hazards associated with the process of decontamination should be minimized. Personnel should be trained to use appropriate personal protective devices and to perform the decontamination in a safe manner.

1. General Procedures

a. All equipment contaminated with potentially infectious materials should be decontaminated prior to cleaning or disposal. Equipment should be cleaned thoroughly prior to storage or re-use. Infectious materials such as cultures of infectious agents and equipment contaminated with these cultures should be sterilized prior to cleaning and/or disposal. The choice of a method of disinfection or sterilization should be based on an evaluation of the specific needs pertinent to the situation.

b. Biohazardous materials should be placed in appropriate containers and properly labeled with the universal biohazard symbol (see Chapter 5, Figure 2). These materials should be decontaminated as soon as is practicable following contamination and should not be left where unsuspecting personnel might come in contact with them.

c. To minimize hazard to firemen or disaster crews, all biohazardous materials should be placed in an appropriately marked refrigerator or incubator, disinfected, sterilized, or otherwise confined at the close of each workday.

d. All personnel should be appropriately trained in the operation of autoclaves to minimize the possibility of improper use, ineffective treatment, and personnel exposure to untreated biohazardous materials.

e. Dry hypochlorite, or any other strong oxidizing material, must not be autoclaved with organic materials such as paper, cloth, or oil: OXIDIZER + ORGANIC MATERIAL + HEAT = EX-PLOSION.
f. Biohazard warning signs (universal biohazard symbol or equivalent) should be used to signify the actual or potential presence of biohazards and to identify equipment, rooms, containers, materials, experimental animals, or combinations of these that contain — or are contaminated with — viable hazardous agents.
g. All work surfaces should be decontaminated at least once a day and after any spill of viable materials.
h. To minimize the entrainment of dust, floors should be swept with push brooms only. The use of floor sweeping compound is recommended because of its effectiveness in limiting the generation of airborne organisms. Vacuum cleaners equipped with filters of an approved type may be used. In all facilities in which infectious agents are used, water used to mop floors should contain an appropriate disinfectant, and should be changed regularly (i.e., every two rooms).
i. Stock solutions of suitable disinfectants should be maintained in each laboratory. If not used immediately, working dilutions should be labeled with the date of dilution and the expiration date.

2. Methods

Physical and chemical means of decontamination fall into four main categories: heat, liquid chemicals, vapors and gases, and radiation. Of these, disinfection is usually limited to liquid chemicals and wet heat (boiling and pasteurization). Wet heat (autoclaving), dry heat, vapors and gases, and radiation are used for sterilization. Some liquid chemicals are also considered sterilants, provided that sufficient time is allowed and the appropriate concentration of the chemical is used.

Heat

Wet heat: Raising the temperature of microbial agents above their normal growth temperature causes a denaturation of their enzymes, resulting in the death of the organism. Organisms vary in their ability to withstand increased temperature, and environmental protein serves to protect the organisms from the effect of the heat.

Boiling: Raising the temperature to 100°C (212°F) and holding for an extended period of time will result in the destruction of most human pathogens but will not kill the spores of bacterial species such as *Bacillus* and *Clostridium*.

Pasteurization: Pasteurization is a heat treatment designed to kill the vegetative cells of any bacteria and fungi, and many viruses. But, again, it will not kill bacterial spores. Some heat-resistant vegetative cells also survive pasteurization.

Two methods of pasteurization generally are used:

- The high temperature/short time (HTST) method, which requires a temperature of 71.7°C (161°F) for a minimum time of 15 seconds; and
- The low temperature/long time (LTLT) method, which requires a temperature of 61.7°C (143°F) for 30 min.

Steam sterilization: Steam sterilization uses pressurized steam at 121–132°C (250–270°F) to kill infectious organisms. Steam sterilization does not substantially reduce waste volume and may increase its weight; therefore, disposal of bulk material remains to be done after treatment. The effectiveness of steam sterilization is a function of temperature and time. Complete removal of air is essential for the steam to completely penetrate the waste and achieve an effective temperature/time exposure. Air removal is affected by type of waste, load density and configuration, and packaging material. In addition to developing a standard operating procedure for steam sterilization, the placement of temperature and biological indicators throughout the load will monitor the effectiveness of the procedure. Temperature indicators change color at specified temperatures. They do not indicate the duration of that temperature or the temperature within enclosed containers. *Bacillus stearothermophilus* is currently the biologic indicator of choice. Spore strips of this organism are commonly placed in the waste and are incubated to determine the effectiveness of a sterilization cycle.

Dry Heat: Dry heat sterilization is less efficient than wet heat sterilization and requires longer times and/or higher temperatures. The specific times and temperatures must be determined for each type of material being sterilized. Generous safety factors are usually added to allow for the variables that can influence the efficiency of this method of sterilization. Sterilization by dry heat can usually be accomplished at 160–170°C (320–338°F) for periods of 2 to 4 hr. Higher temperatures and shorter times may be used for heat-resistant materials. The heat transfer properties and the spatial relation or arrangement of articles in the load are critical in ensuring effective sterilization.

Liquid Disinfection/Sterilization

The appropriate liquid disinfectant should be chosen following careful consideration of the potential contamination present, and the type of material to be decontaminated. Liquid disinfectants are most useful for the decontamination of solid surfaces and equipment. Some may be used for the decontamination of liquid waste, provided that the appropriate concentrations are used. A disinfectant with "tuberculocidal" properties should be used if a general "all-purpose" disinfectant is needed.

Remember that most chemical disinfectants are not sterilizers and should not be relied on to destroy all organisms on a surface or piece of equipment. Simple wiping of the surface to be decontaminated with a liquid disinfectant does not kill the organisms present. Chemical disinfectants cause inactivation of organisms either by coagulation and denaturation of proteins; lysis; or inactivation of an essential enzyme system by oxidation, binding, or destruction of the enzyme substrate; therefore, factors such as time, pH, concentration, temperature, and the amount and type of organic material all affect the activity of these agents.

Liquid disinfectants should always be used in accordance with the manufacturer's recommendations. Failure to follow instructions might result in an inactive or ineffective material.

There are many liquid disinfectants available under a wide variety of trade names. In general, these can be categorized as halogens, acids or alkalies, heavy metal salts, quaternary ammonium compounds, phenolic compounds, aldehydes, ketones, alcohols, and amines. Unfortunately, the more active disinfectants often possess undesirable characteristics, such as corrosive properties. None is equally useful or effective under all conditions.

Alcohols: Ethyl or isopropyl alcohol in concentrations of 70%–95% are good general-use disinfectants. They are active against lipid-containing viruses but are much less active against nonlipid viruses and are not effective against bacterial spores. Alcohols act to denature proteins but are not so caustic as to be significantly harmful to personnel using them. Care should be taken not to use alcohols near open flames since they are flammable at the use dilutions.

Formalin: Formalin is a 37% solution of formaldehyde in water. Diluted to 5% active ingredient formalin is an effective disinfectant. At concentrations of 0.2%–0.4% it is used to inactivate bacteria and viruses, and it acts as a preservative in vaccine production. Formalin has a pungent, irritating odor, and personnel exposure must be limited because of its toxicity and potential carcinogenicity.

Glutaraldehydes: These agents are closely related to formaldehyde but seem to be more biologically active. Both alkaline and acidic forms of glutaraldehyde have been developed for use as disinfectants. The glutaraldehydes are active against all types of bacteria, fungi, and viruses. When used for extended periods, they can be used as sterilants since they kill bacterial spores. The glutaraldehydes are used primarily for disinfection and sterilization of equipment and medical devices.

Glutaraldehyde disinfectants should always be used in accordance with the manufacturer's directions. Vapors of glutaraldehyde are known to be severely irritating to the eyes, nasal passages, and upper respiratory tract. These agents should be used in well-ventilated areas, and personnel should be provided with appropriate personal protective devices to prevent exposure.

Phenol and phenol derivatives: Solutions of 5% phenol in water have been used for many years as a disinfectant. Phenol solutions have a strong, somewhat unpleasant odor and a sticky residue is left on surfaces following treatment with this material. Phenol is quite toxic. Personnel using this material should be appropriately protected from skin exposure.

Phenol activity has been the standard by which the activity of other disinfectants has been compared. Care must be taken in this comparison, however, since the activity of phenol is significantly different from the activity of other non-phenol based disinfectant agents and comparison of phenol to these disinfectants is not always valid.

Phenol homologs and other phenolic-based compounds have become popular disinfectants. These are recommended for the killing of vegetative bacteria, including *Mycobacterium tuberculosis*, fungi, and lipid-containing viruses. They are not active against bacterial spores and nonlipid-containing viruses. The phenolic disinfectants are used most commonly for cleaning and disinfection of contaminated surfaces (i.e., walls, floors, bench tops).

Quaternary Ammonium Compounds (Quats): Quats are cationic detergents and are strong surface active agents. They are acceptable for general-use disinfectants and are active against vegetative Gram-positive bacteria and lipid-containing viruses. The quats are less active against Gram-negative bacteria and are not active against nonlipid-containing viruses at normal use dilutions. These agents are also not active against bacterial spores.

Quaternary ammonium compounds are easily inactivated by the presence of excess organic material, anionic detergents, and the salts of metals found in water. Some bacteria, notably *Pseudomonas* strains have been found growing in dilute solutions of these disinfectants. Mixtures of quats and phenol-based anionic detergent solutions may result in total inactivation of both agents.

Quats are relatively nontoxic and can be used for decontamination of food equipment and for general cleaning.

Halogens (Chlorine and Iodine): Chlorine-containing solutions have universal disinfectant activity. Sodium hypochlorite is the usual base for chlorine disinfectants. Household or laundry bleach (5.25% available chlorine) can be diluted 1/100 with water to yield a disinfectant solution containing 525 ppm of available chlorine. Diluted solutions may be kept for extended periods of time with little loss of activity, provided that the solution is kept in a stoppered bottle and protected from light. This material is active against a wide variety of bacteria, fungi, and viruses. At higher concentrations with extended contacttimes, hypochlorite solutions can be considered chemical sterilants since they will inactivate bacterial spores.

Chlorine-containing disinfectants are inactivated by excess organic materials and little or no residual activity remains after use. Chlorine and chlorine-containing solutions are strong oxidizing agents and are corrosive to metals and tissues. Appropriate precautions should be taken by personnel working with these agents.

Iodine solution has long been used as a disinfectant and antiseptic. Iodine has many of the same properties of chlorine with regard to antimicrobial activity. Iodophors (organically bound iodine) are recommended as disinfectants. They have a relatively broad range of activity, being active against all vegetative forms of bacteria, fungi, and viruses. These agents are relatively nontoxic to humans and therefore have been used as antiseptics and in surgical soaps. Small amounts of organic material might inactivate them.

Pertinent characteristics and potential applications for several categories of chemical disinfectants most likely to be used in the biological laboratory are summarized in Tables XXIII–XXVI. Practical concentrations and contact times that may differ markedly from the recommendations of manufacturers of proprietary products are suggested. It has been presumed that microorganisms will be afforded a high degree of potential protection by organic menstruums. It has not been presumed that a sterile state will result from application of the indicated concentrations and contact times. It should be emphasized that these data are only indicative of efficacy under artificial test conditions. The efficacy of any of the disinfectants should be determined conclusively by individual investigators. It is readily evident that each of the disinfectants has a range of advantages and disadvantages in addition to a range of potential for inactivation of a diverse microflora. Equally evident is the need for compromise as an alternative to maintaining a veritable "drug store" of disinfectants.

Table XXIII. Summary of Practical Disinfectants

Disinfectants		Practical Requirements					Inactivates			
			Contact Time (min.)							
Type	Category	Use Dilution	Lipovirus	Broad Spectrum	Temperature (°C)	Relative Humidity (%)	Vegetative Bacteria	Lipoviruses	Nonlipid Viruses	Bacterial Spores
Liquid	Quat. Ammon. Cpds	0.1%–2.0%	10	NE [A]			+	+		
	Phenolic Cpds	1.0%–5.0%	10	NE			+	+	[B]	
	Chlorine Cpds	500 ppm [C]	10	30			+	+	+	+

104

	Iodophor	25–1600 ppm [c]	10	30				+	+	+	+
	Alcohol, Ethyl	70%–85%	10	NE				+	+	[B]	
	Alcohol, Isopropyl	70%–85%	10	NE				+	+	[B]	
	Formaldehyde	0.2%–8.0%	10	30				+	+	+	+
	Gluteraldehyde	2%	10	30				+	+	+	+
Gas	Ethylene Oxide	8–23 g/ft³	60	60	37	30		+	+	+	+
	Paraformaldehyde	0.3 g/ft³	60	60	> 23	> 60		+	+	+	+

[A] NE = not effective

[B] variable results dependent on virus

[C] available halogen

Table XXIV. Summary of Practical Disinfectants

Disinfectants		Important Characteristics										
Type	Category	Effective Shelf Life > 1 week [A]	Corrosive	Flammable	Explosion Potential	Residue	Inactivated by Organic Matter	Compatible for Optics [D]	Compatible for Electronics	Skin Irritant	Eye Irritant	Respiratory Irritant / Toxic [E]
Liquid												
	Quat. Ammon. Cpds	+					+	+		+	+	+
	Phenolic Cpds	+	+		+					+	+	+
	Chlorine Cpds		+		+	+				+	+	+ +
	Iodophor	+	+		+	+				+	+	+
	Alcohol, Ethyl	+		+							+	+
	Alcohol, Isopropyl	+		+							+	+
	Formaldehyde	+			+					+	+	+
	Gluteraldehyde	+			+		+			+	+	+
Gas												
	Ethylene Oxide	N/A		+ [B]	+ [B]			+	+	+	+	+ +
	Paraformaldehyde	N/A		+ [C]	+ [C]			+	+	+	+	+ +

N/A = not applicable.

[A] protected from light and air.

[B] neither flammable nor explosive in 90% CO_2 or fluorinate hydrocarbon, the usual use form.

[C] at concentrations of 7%–73% by volume in air, solid-exposure to open flame.

[D] Usually compatible, but consider interferences from residues and effects on associated materials such as mounting adhesives.

[E] By skin or mouth, or both. Refer to manufacturer's literature and/or *The Merck Index*.

Table XV. Summary of Practical Disinfectants

Disinfectants		Potential Application										
Type	Category	Work Surfaces	Dirty Glassware	Large Area Decon.	Air Handling Systems	Portable Equip. Surface Decon.	Portable Equip. Penetrat-ing Decon.	Fixed Equip. Surface Decon.	Fixed Equip. Penetrat-ing Decon	Optical & Electronic Instruments	Liquids for Discard	Books, Papers
Liquid												
	Quat. Ammon. Cpds	+	+			+		+				

	C1	C2	C3	C4	C5	C6	C7	C8	C9	C10	C11
Phenolic Cpds	+	+			+		+				
Chlorine Cpds	+	+			+		+			+	
Iodophor	+	+			+		+				
Alcohol, Ethyl	+	+			+		+				
Alcohol, Isopropyl	+	+			+		+				
Formaldehyde	+	+			+		+				
Gluteraldehyde	+	+			+		+				
Gas											
Ethylene Oxide						+			+		+
Paraformaldehyde			+	+		+		+	+		

Table XXVI. Summary of Practical Disinfectants

Disinfectants Type	Category	Examples of Proprietary Disinfectants [A]
Liquid	Quat. Ammon. Cpds	A-33, CDQ, End-Bac, Hi-Tor, Mikro-Quat
	Phenolic Cpds	Hil-Phene, Matar, Midro-Bac, O-Syl
	Chlorine Cpds	Chloramine T, Clorox, Purex
	Iodophor	Hy-Sine, Ioprep, Mikroklene, Wescodyne
	Alcohol, Ethyl	N/A
	Alcohol, Isopropyl	N/A
	Formaldehyde	Sterac
	Gluteraldehyde	Cidex
Gas	Ethylene	Carboxide, Cryoxicide, Steroxicide
	Paraformaldehyde	—

N/A = not applicable

[A] Space limitations preclude listing all products available. Individual listings (or omissions) do not imply endorsement or rejection of any product by the National Institutes of Health.

Vapors and Gases

A variety of vapors and gases possess germicidal properties. The most useful of these are formaldehyde and ethylene oxide. When these are used in closed systems and under controlled conditions of temperature and humidity, sterilization can be achieved. Vapor and gas disinfectants are primarily useful in sterilizing 1) biological safety cabinets and associated effluent air-handling systems and air filters; 2) bulky or stationary equipment that resists penetration by liquid surface disinfectants; 3) instruments and optics that might be damaged by other sterilization methods; and 4) rooms and buildings and associated air-handling systems.

Other chemical disinfectants used as space decontaminants include peracetic acid, betapropiolactone (BPL), methyl bromide and glutaraldehyde. These are excellent disinfectants when used in closed systems and under controlled conditions of temperature and humidity. Peracetic acid is a fast-acting, universal germicide. In the concentrated state, however, it is a hazardous compound that can readily decompose with explosive violence. When diluted for use, it has a short half-life, produces strong, pungent, irritating odors, and is extremely corrosive to metals. Nevertheless, it is such an outstanding germicide that it is commonly used in germ-free animal studies despite these undesirable characteristics. Peracetic acid is corrosive to metals and rubber. BPL is not recommended as a space disinfectant since it is listed as a carcinogen by OSHA (*Federal Register 39:*20 [20 January 1974]).

Formaldehyde: Formaldehyde, in general, is the chemical of choice for space disinfection. Safety cabinets, incubators, laboratory rooms, buildings, or other enclosed spaces can be disinfected with formaldehyde. The formaldehyde can be generated from aqueous solutions (formalin) containing 37%–40% formaldehyde by heating or by vaporizing the solution. Formaldehyde gas can also be generated by heating paraformaldehyde, which is a solid polymer that contains 91%–99% formaldehyde. If aqueous formaldehyde is used, the application rate should be 1 mL for each cubic foot of space to be treated. Also, if a small amount of exhaust air is used to keep the area being treated under a slightly reduced pressure, then this amount must be known, and 1 mL of formalin added for each cubic foot of exhaust air for at least a one-hour period. To assure thorough mixing, the use of air-circulating fans may be required. Areas being treated should have a temperature of at least 21°C (70°F) and a relative humidity above 70 percent. Spaces being treated should not be wet, have condensate on the walls, or have pools of water on the floor since formaldehyde is quite soluble in water and will be taken up rapidly. Also, as the water evaporates, polymerization will take place on the surfaces, and these polymers are difficult to remove. Formaldehyde is a powerful reducing agent and is noncorrosive to metals. It can normally be presumed that any equipment or apparatus that will not be damaged by the humidity necessary for decontamination will not be damaged by the formaldehyde. Although formaldehyde will sterilize all exposed surfaces, it has limited penetrating abilities; materials that are tightly covered might not be sterilized. This lack of penetrating power is often an advantage in using formaldehyde since the space only needs to be enclosed relatively tightly instead of hermetically sealed — a condition impossible to achieve when rooms or buildings are being treated.

Generally, the generation of formaldehyde gas from powdered or flake paraformaldehyde by heating is the preferred method. Paraformaldehyde will depolymerize and convert to the gaseous state when heated to a temperature above 150°C (302°F). A concentration of 0.3 g of paraformaldehyde for each cubic foot of space to be treated is used. Temperature of the space must be above 20°C (38°F) and relative humidity must be 70% or higher. Exposure times should be at least two hours and, if possible, the exposure should be for eight hours or overnight. Formaldehyde generated from paraformaldehyde has better penetration and fewer problems with condensation and subsequent need for prolonged aeration than with formaldehyde generated from formalin. If walls and surfaces were not wet with condensation during the formaldehyde treatment process, then aeration and removal of the formaldehyde should proceed rapidly. A small room with nonporous surfaces and no materials or equipment in the room can be cleared of all detectable formaldehyde in less than an hour of aeration; however, an entire building containing a variety of surfaces and equipment may take many hours or even a day or more of aeration to remove the formaldehyde.

Formaldehyde, a toxic substance and a suspected human carcinogen, is regulated by OSHA. Considerable caution must be exercised in handling, storing, and using formaldehyde. Repeated exposure to formaldehyde is known to produce a hypersensitive condition in certain individuals. Self-contained breathing apparatus, air-supplied masks, or industrial-type gas masks should be available and used whenever exposure to formaldehyde is possible. Most individuals can readily detect formaldehyde at a concentration of 1 ppm, which serves as a warning to avoid excessive exposure. Chemicals, such as anhydrous ammonia, have been used to neutralize formaldehyde and deposited paraformaldehyde with limited success. Air containing formaldehyde can be passed through alumina to adsorb the formaldehyde. This technique is useful in removing formaldehyde from cabinets and other small places, but impractical quantities of alumina are required for removing the formaldehyde from large rooms or buildings. Recent reports indicate that formaldehyde may combine with hydrochloric acid to form bis(chloromethyl)ether, a carcinogenic compound. When formaldehyde is to be used as a space disinfectant, the area to be treated should be surveyed to ensure that there are no open containers of any acidic solution containing chloride ion. Note that formaldehyde in the concentrations used for space disinfection has no effect on cockroaches and possibly not on other insects or arachnids.

Formaldehyde is explosive at concentrations between 7.0% and 73.0% by volume in air. This concentration, however, cannot be reached when standard procedures for disinfection are used.

Ethylene Oxide Sterilization: Ethylene oxide (EtO) gas is lethal for microorganisms, including spores, viruses, molds, pathogenic fungi, and highly resistant thermophilic bacteria. Following are some of the principal variables that determine the rate microorganisms will be destroyed by ethylene oxide:

- *Temperature:* Temperature affects the penetration of EtO through microbial cell walls and wrapping and/or packaging materials. The activity of ethylene oxide will increase approximately 2.7 times for each 10°C (18°F) rise in temperature [between ranges of 5°C and 37°C (41°F and 98.6°F) using a concentration of 884 mg/L]. Normally, EtO sterilization is conducted at temperatures between 49°C and 60°C (120° and 140°F).
- *Ethylene Oxide Concentration:* Sterilization with EtO can be achieved in shorter periods when the concentration is increased. For practical sterilization, gas concentrations of 500 to 1000 mg/L at approximately 49–60°C (120–140°F) are recommended.
- *Humidity:* It is generally accepted that moisture is an essential condition in achieving sterilization with EtO gas. The effect of moisture on the sterilizing action of ethylene oxide seems to be related to the moisture content of the exposed bacterial cells. A relative humidity of 30%–60% frequently is used in EtO chambers during such exposure conditions.
- *Exposure Time:* In most cases, the appropriate exposure time for attaining sterility is determined experimentally using accepted biological indicators. Frequently, these controls are *Bacillus subtilis* var. *niger* spores placed on suitable carrier materials.
- *Precautions in Using Ethylene Oxide:* Ethylene oxide is a human carcinogen and regulated by OSHA. Its concentration must be monitored when used. During treatment, it is absorbed by certain items; therefore all clothing, shoes, masks, adhesive tape, and other items designated for contact with human skin should be exposed to circulating air for at least 25 hours after sterilization with EtO and prior to use. This precaution is particularly important with rubber articles. If the air is cold, the aeration time must be increased. Mixtures of 3%–10% ethylene oxide in air are explosive. Commercially available mixtures of EtO in Freon® or CO_2 are not explosive and can be used safely.

Radiation: Gamma and X-ray are the two principle types of ionizing radiation used in sterilization for their activity against bacteria, spores, and viruses. Ionizing radiation is usually recommended for the sterilization of prepackaged medical devices, including syringes and catheters. Caution should be used in selecting the type of material for ionizing radiation sterilization: Polypropylene tends to become brittle, PVC discolors, and cotton loses tensile strength. In most cases, ionizing radiation is not a practical tool for laboratory use.

Ultraviolet (UV) radiation is a practical method for inactivating viruses, mycoplasma, bacteria, and fungi. This nonionizing radiation is especially useful for the destruction of airborne microorganisms and, to a lesser extent, for the inactivation of microorganisms on exposed surfaces or for the treatment of products of unstable composition that cannot be treated by conventional methods. The usefulness of ultraviolet radiation as a sanitizer is limited by its low penetrating power. Ultraviolet light is primarily useful in air locks, animal holding areas, ventilated cabinets, and in laboratory rooms during periods of nonoccupancy to reduce the level of viable airborne microorganisms and to maintain good air hygiene.

Sterilization

General criteria for sterilization of typical materials are presented below. It is advised to review the type of materials being handled and to establishstandard conditions for sterilization. Treatment conditions to achieve sterility will vary in relation to the volume of material treated, its contamination level, the moisture content, and other factors.

Steam Autoclave:
1. *Laundry:* 121°C (250°F) for 30 min with 15 min prevacuum of 27 inches of mercury (in. Hg.)
2. *Trash:* 121°C (250°F) for 1 hr with 15 min prevacuum of 27 in. Hg.
3. *Glassware:* 121°C (250°F) for 1 hr with 15 min prevacuum of 27 in. Hg.
4. *Liquids:* 121°C (250°F) for 1 hr for each gallon
5. *Animals:* 121°C (250°F) for 8 hr with 15 min prevacuum of 27 in. Hg.
6. *Bedding:* 121°C (250°F) for 8 hr with 15 min prevacuum of 27 in. Hg.

Gas Sterilants:
1. *Ethylene oxide gas* — Sixteen hours exposure to a concentration of 750 mg/L (±5%) at 30%–60% relative humidity and at ambient temperatures (>70°F).

2. *Paraformaldehyde* — Sixteen hours exposure to a concentration of 1.0 mg/L at 40%–60% humidity and at ambient temperatures (>70°F).

Liquid Sterilants:
1. *Mercurials* — Not recommended for general use because they have poor activity against vegetative bacteria and are useless as sporicides. Although the mercurials exhibit good activity against viruses (1:500 to 1:1000 concentration), they are toxic and therefore not recommended.
2. *Quaternary Ammonium Compounds* — These are acceptable as general-use disinfectants to control vegetative bacteria and nonlipid-containing viruses; however, they are not active against bacterial spores at the usual use concentrations (1:750).
3. *Phenolic Compounds* — These are recommended for the killing of vegetative bacteria, including *Mycobacterium tuberculosis*, fungi, and lipid-containing viruses (0.5%–2.0%). They are less effective against spores and nonlipid-containing viruses.
4. *Chlorine Compounds* — These are recommended for certain disinfecting procedures, provided that the available chlorine needed is considered. Low concentrations of available chlorine (50–500 ppm) are active against vegetative bacteria and most viruses. For bacterial spores, concentrations of approximately 2500 ppm are needed. The corrosive nature of these compounds, their decay rates, and lack of residuals is such that they are recommended only in special situations.
5. *Iodophors* — Although these show poor activity against bacterial spores, they are recommended for general use (75–150 ppm). They are effective against vegetative bacteria and viruses. Their advantages are:

   – Iodophors possess a wide spectrum of antimicrobial and antiviral activity.
   – Iodophors have a built-in indicator. If the solution is brown or yellow, it is still active.
   – Iodophors are relatively harmless to man.
   – Iodophors can be readily inactivated, and iodophor stains can be readily removed with solutions of $Na_2S_2O_3$ (sodium thiosulfate).

6. *Alcohols* — In concentrations of 70%–95%, alcoholic solutions are good general-use disinfectants, but they exhibit no activity against bacterial spores.
7. *Formaldehyde Solutions* — At concentrations of 8%, formalin exhibits good activity against vegetative bacteria, spores, and viruses.
8. *Formaldehyde-Alcohol* — Solutions of 8% formalin in 70% alcohol are considered very good for disinfection purposes because of their effectiveness against vegetative bacteria, spores, and viruses. For many applications, this is the disinfectant of choice.

Ionizing Radiation: A dose of 25 Gy (2.5 mrad) is generally accepted as effective for sterilization.

3. Precautions for Applying Decontamination Methods

Heat Sterilization — The hazards of handling hot solids and liquids are reasonably familiar. Laboratory personnel should be cautioned that steam under pressure can be a source of scalding jets if the equipment for its application is mishandled. Loads of manageable size should be used. Fluids treated by steam under pressure may be superheated if removed from the sterilizer too promptly after treatment. This can cause a sudden and violent boiling of the contents from containers that can splash scalding liquids onto personnel handling the containers.

Liquid Disinfectants — Particular care should be observed when handling concentrated stock solutions of disinfectants. Personnel assigned the task of making up use-concentrations from stock solutions must be properly informed of potential hazards and trained in the safe procedures to follow. The concentrated quaternary and phenolic disinfectants are particularly harmful to the eyes. Even a small droplet splashed in the eyes may cause blindness. Protective face shields and goggles should be used for eye protection, and long-sleeved garments and chemically resistant gloves, aprons, and boots should be worn to protect from corrosive and depigmentation effects to the skin. One of the initial sources for hazard information on any given product will be the label on its container.

Vapors and Gases — Avoid inhalation of vapors of formaldehyde and ethylene oxide. Stock containers of these products should be capable of containing these vapors and should be kept in properly ventilated chemical storage areas in the event of inadvertent leakage. In preparing use-dilutions and when applying them, personnel should control the operations to prevent exposure of others and wear respiratory protection as necessary. Mutagenic potential has been attributed to ethylene oxide; toxic and hypersensitivity effects are well-established for formaldehyde.

Radiation — The uses of UV irradiation carry the danger of burns to the cornea of the eyes and the skin of persons exposed for even a short period. Proper shielding should be maintained where irradiation treatment is used when personnel and laboratory animals are present. Guard against reflecting surfaces (e.g., polished stainless steel) occurring in line with the light source. In areas irradiated without shielding on special occasions or during off-duty hours, post the area with warning signs to prevent unscheduled entry of personnel.

Ionizing Radiation — Irradiators should be purchased through a supplier licensed by the Nuclear Regulatory Commission (NRC) or the state. Employees should be trained in the properties of ionizing radiation and emergency procedures. Proper warnings and labels must be installed in the irradiator's location. Wipe tests intended to ensure source integrity should be conducted routinely.

4. Summary

Disinfectants are used to reduce the number of pathogenic organisms present in or on contaminated materials. There is no single disinfectant that can be used for all circumstances; therefore, the choice of a disinfectant should be made after careful consideration of a number of factors. These factors would include: 1) the number and type of organisms possibly present; 2) the amount of extraneous organic material present; 3) the material to be decontaminated; 4) the potential toxicity of the disinfectant; and 5) the activity of the disinfectant.

Disinfectants should always be used in accordance with the manufacturer's directions. Failure to do so will result in failure of the disinfectant to perform appropriately. Personnel assigned to use these agents should be fully informed of the proper methods of application, and of the hazards associated with their use.

Disinfectants are designed to kill living cells by interacting with the cells and disrupting their metabolism. As such they are toxic, not only to the organisms they are designed to kill but also to those individuals who must use them. Appropriate precautions must be taken by all personnel using disinfectants in order to minimize exposure to these agents.

B. Infectious Waste Decontamination and Disposal

The term "infectious waste" includes substances capable of causing an infectious disease. The risk associated with this waste is a function of the virulence of the contaminating organisms, their concentration, the route of exposure, and host susceptibility.

Infectious waste is generated in a variety of health care institutions; the food, drug, cosmetic, and biotechnology industries; and research laboratories.

Infectious waste is generated from a variety of materials including but not limited to:
- waste from patients isolated to protect others from communicable disease;
- cultures and stocks of infectious agents discarded from laboratories culturing specimens from patients or doing research using human pathogens;
- human blood and blood products;
- pathologic waste removed during biopsy, surgery, or autopsy;
- waste generated from surgical or autopsy procedures of patients with infectious disease, including disposable supplies, equipment, and patient dressings and drapes;
- waste generated in laboratories involved with pathogenic organisms;
- contaminated sharps, including discarded hypodermic needles, syringes, pipettes, broken glassware, and scalpel blades;
- dialysis unit waste;
- contaminated animal waste, carcasses, and bedding; and
- contaminated food.

Decontamination and disposal of infectious waste are closely interrelated acts in which disinfection constitutes the first phase of disposal. Disposal should therefore be interpreted in the broadest sense of the word, rather than in the restrictive sense of dealing solely with a destructive process.

Laboratory materials requiring disposal will normally occur as liquid, solid, and animal room wastes. The volume of these can become a major problem when there is the requirement that all waste be disinfected prior to disposal. It is most evident that a significant portion of this problem can be eliminated if the kinds of materials initially entering the laboratory are reduced. In any case, and wherever possible, nonessential materials should be retained in the noncontamination areas for disposal by conventional methods. Examples are the packaging materials in which goods are delivered, disposable carton-cages for transport of animals, and large carboys or tanks of fluids that can be left outside and drawn from as required. Reduction of this bulk will free autoclaves and other decontamination and disposal processes within the laboratory for more rapid and efficient handling of materials known to be contaminated.

Noninfectious materials of dissimilar nature will be common in facilities with infectious waste. Examples are combinations of common flammable solvents, chemical carcinogens, and radioactive isotopes. These may require input from a number of disciplines in arriving at the most practical approach for their decontamination and disposal.

Disposal of infectious waste will be required for research projects ranging in size from an individual researcher to those involving large numbers of researchers of many disciplines. Procedures and facilities to accomplish this will range from the simplest to the most elaborate. The primary consideration in any case is to dispel the notion that laboratory wastes can be disposed of in the same manner, and with as little thought, as household wastes. Selection and enforcement of safe procedures for disposal of laboratory materials are of no less importance than the consideration given to any other methodology for the accomplishment of research objectives or the mission of the facility.

The principal questions to be answered prior to disposal of any objects or materials from facilities dealing with potentially infectious microorganisms or animal tissues are:

- Have the objects or materials been effectively disinfected or sterilized by an approved procedure?

Two methods are generally used to treat infectious waste: incineration and sterilization (see previous section). Incineration relies on high temperature combustion to render waste noninfective. There are three types of incinerators:

1. The single chamber, "type 4," or "pathological" incinerator operates at a temperature of 1200–1400°F (649–760°C). This type of incinerator is suitable for pathologic waste but not for chemotherapy waste or waste-containing plastics.
2. The single-chamber incinerator with an afterburner operates at a temperature of 1600–1800°F (871–982°C). An afterburner is located in the incinerator stack, allowing for additional incineration or combustion of gases.
3. The two-chambered controlled-air incinerator burns waste at a reduced air concentration in the primary chamber (1600–1800°F) followed by excess air combustion in the secondary chamber (2000–2200°F [1093–1204°C]). Gas retention in the secondary chamber ranges from a minimum of 0.5 seconds.

- If the objects have not been effectively disinfected or sterilized by an approved procedure, have the objects or materials been packaged in an approved manner for immediate on-site incineration or transfer to another laboratory?

The type of container used to package infectious waste depends on the type of waste, methods of handling and moving the waste, storage conditions, and type of treatment. The most commonly used containers for nonsharp, nonwet waste are the plastic red or orange biohazard bags. These colors are universally recognized for biohazardous materials and are tearproof and leakproof. For liquids waste, primary leakproof containers enclosed either in an outer leakproof container or an outer container with an absorbent packing material are necessary to prevent spills or leaks during transport and handling. For discarded syringe needles, scalpels, broken glass, etc., special rigid plastic containers should be available in each facility to minimize the handling of untreated sharps.

Containers of infectious waste should be readily identifiable by special labels or markings. Special colors, symbols, or wording should be placed directly on the waste container. If the containers are to be reused, then labels must be removed prior to reuse of the container. For transport, each container must be appropriately labeled. The name, address, and telephone number of the waste generator, the waste hauler, and the treatment facility must be included. The appropriate emergency contact must also be designated on the container in case of an accident or spill. If infectious waste is to be stored prior to treatment, storage conditions should be designed to minimize the potential for employee exposure and to prevent the amplification of the infectious potential of the waste. Storage areas should be clearly identified with signs, and entry should be limited to trained personnel. Storage areas should be cleaned and disinfected regularly and should be free of vermin to prevent vector borne transmission.

- Does disposal of the disinfected or sterilized objects or materials involve any additional potential hazards, biological or otherwise, to those carrying out the immediate disposal procedures or those who might come into contact with the objects or materials outside the laboratory complex?

Inevitably, disposal of materials raises the question: "How can we be sure that the materials have been treated adequately to ensure that their disposal does not constitute a hazard?" In the small laboratory, the problem is often solved by having each investigator disinfect all contaminated materials not of immediate use at the end of each day and place them in suitable containers for routine disposal. In larger laboratories, where the mass of materials for disposal becomes much greater and sterilization bottlenecks occur, materials handling and disposal will likely be the chore of personnel not engaged in the actual research. In either situation, an infectious waste management program is necessary to assure that the waste is handled, rendered noninfectious, and disposed of safely. The elements of an effective infectious waste management program include:

- identification of the type of infectious waste;
- segregation of the infectious waste from noninfectious waste at the point of waste generation;
- appropriate packaging and labeling of the waste;
- handling and moving the waste both before and after treatment;
- waste storage before and after treatment; and
- waste treatment.

No federal regulations apply to infectious waste. The Resource Conservation and Recovery Act (RCRA 1976), the Comprehensive Environmental Response, Compensation, and Liability Act (CERCLA 1980), and their amendments — the Hazardous and Solid Waste Amendments (1984) and the Superfund Amendments and Reauthorization Act of 1986 (SARA) — give the U.S. Environmental Protection Agency the authority to regulate hazardous waste disposal. The EPA has discussed the regulation of infectious waste as a hazardous waste and has issued two guidance manuals on its management, but to date it has not issued specific regulations. Under RCRA, however, the states have the authority to regulate hazardous waste, and several have issued regulations specific for infectious waste.

Also, the U.S. Congress passed the Medical Waste Tracking Act of 1988 in response to medical waste on beaches along the Atlantic coast. This act required the EPA to determine the effectiveness of tracking regulations through a two-year tracking program. In 1989, the EPA issued the medical waste tracking regulation applicable to certain types of medical waste. It imposed packaging requirements and required tracking from point of generation to disposal. The regulations applied specifically to several states in the Northeast and to Puerto Rico. In a December 1990 interim report to Congress on the Medical Waste Tracking Act, the EPA made no conclusions about the demonstration program's effectiveness. The EPA suggested that the findings of the act could lead to development of model practices for regulating medical waste in communities.[1]

C. Emergency Response for Spills of Infectious Waste

Spills of infectious waste can occur in facilities that generate infectious and medical waste, and in the transportation and disposal of that waste, and emergency response procedures are necessary for managing such events. These procedures must be developed as part of a comprehensive program of biosafety and be in place before they are needed. Planning for emergencies requires a systematic approach that consists of anticipating possible incidents, developing procedures and practices to prevent their occurrence, and defining the responses in case these incidents occur.

Emergency response for chemical hazards is covered by Title III of the Superfund Amendments and Reauthorization Act. Under SARA requirements, facilities using any listed chemical hazardous substance above a designated threshold quantity must notify the local emergency planning committee, the state emergency response commission, and the local fire department. Although many research and medical facilities do not meet the threshold planning quantity levels, those exceeding the threshold levels must develop contingency plans as published in the Code of Federal Regulations (40 CFR 262.34(d)(5)); however, emergency planning for spills of infectious agents or other biogenic substances are not regulated at the federal level.

Although there may be standards or guidance issued by accrediting bodies or through nonmandatory planning efforts by individual institutions, there is no single guideline or standard that applies to emergency planning for infections agents. Until such guidelines are available, each institution must develop and tailor an emergency response plan to its specific needs. The components of an emergency response plan include:

1. Anticipating the Hazard (Infectious Agent)
    a. Analysis of infectious, allergenic, or toxic materials, and how they are stored, used (including potential routes of exposure), and disposed of.
    b. Analysis of work practices or laboratory procedures.
    c. Analysis of equipment safety and containment design and efficacy of equipment, cabinets, and PPE as primary barriers.
    d. Analysis of the secondary barrier properties of the facility.
2. Post-Anticipation Prevention
    a. *Engineering Controls* — Assure that engineering controls are in place and routinely evaluated for proper operation.
    b. *Contingency Plan* — A model for a written contingency plan for hazardous substances, as proposed by the federal National Response Team, is shown in Table XXVII (Hazardous Materials Emergency Planning Guide, National Response Team, NRT-1 [March 1987]).

Table XXVII. Components of a Sample Hazardous Materials Emergency Plan

A. Introduction
    1. Incident information summary
    2. Promulgation document
    3. Legal authority and responsibility for responding
    4. Table of contents
    5. Abbreviations and definitions
    6. Assumptions/planning factors
    7. Concept of operations
       a. Governing Principles
       b. Organizational roles and responsibilities
       c. Relationship to other plans
    8. Instructions on plan use
       a. Purpose
       b. Plan distribution
    9. Record of amendments

B. Emergency assistance telephone roster

C. Response functions
    1. Initial notification of response agencies
    2. Direction and control
    3. Communications (among responders)
    4. Warning systems and emergency public notification
    5. Public information/community relations
    6. Resource management
    7. Health and medical services
    8. Response personnel safety
    9. Personal protection of citizens
       a. Indoor protection
       b. Evacuation procedures
       c. Other public protection strategies
    10. Fire and rescue
    11. Law enforcement
    12. Ongoing incident assessment

13. Human services
14. Public works
15. Others

D. Containment and cleanup
  1. Techniques for spill containment and cleanup
  2. Resources for cleanup and disposal

E. Documentation and investigative follow-up

F. Procedures for testing and updating plan
  1. Testing the plan
  2. Updating the plan

G. Hazards analysis (summary)

H. References
  1. Laboratory, consultant, and other technical support resources
  2. Technical library

---

  i.   Identify an emergency response coordinator.
  ii.   Establish a hierarchy of command and define lines of communication.
  iii. Develop an emergency response plan (contingency plan) that addresses only those incidences with the highest probability of occurrence. Such a plan should include:

  – development of containment and cleanup procedures for different categories of infectious waste, for waste containing multiple biohazards, and for waste with unknown biohazards;
  – identification and assignment of persons responsible for the cleanup; assignments should be based on the type of waste, area in the facility at risk, and training and skills of the personnel;
  – Placement of cleanup equipment and personal protective equipment in easily accessible locations; and
  – specific procedures for accident reports, accident assessment, corrective action, and follow-up should be developed.

  iv.   Train employees annually in the safe handling of biohazards and in emergency response procedures.

  c. *Communication Controls* — Assure that the internal communication necessary to warn for evacuation (e.g., alarms) is operational and evaluated on a routine basis; that external communication for contacting outside responders is available and operational; and that appropriate phone numbers are available.
  d. *Primary Prevention and Medical Surveillance* — When appropriate, administer immunizations (e.g., hepatitis B) and establish a routine medical surveillance program to monitor worker health (see Chapter 5: Control Methods).
  3. Emergency Response (implementation of the contingency plan).

References

1. **U.S. Environmental Protection Agency:** *EPA Guide for Infectious Waste Management* (EPA Document #530-SW-86-014). Springfield, Va.: National Technical Information Service, May 1986.

Appendix I

Bibliography

The literature sources in this bibliography have not been cited specifically in the main text but are useful in providing a more in-depth look at important areas in the broad field of biosafety. The second part of this bibliography includes a list of significant bioaerosol sampling documents.

Adams, R.M.: *Occupational Contact Dermatitis.* Philadelphia: J.B. Lippincott Co., 1969.

al-Alska, A.K., and A.H. Chagla: Laboratory-Acquired Brucellosis. *J. Hosp. Infect. 14(1):*69-71 (1989).

Aly, R., H. Mailbach, and E. Bloom: Quantification of Anaerobic Diptheroids on the Skin. *Acta Dermatoveuer 58:*501-504 (1978).

American Society of Heating, Refrigerating and Air-Conditioning Engineers: *ASHRAE Handbook and Product Directory: 1978 Applications.* New York: American Society of Heating, Refrigerating and Air-Conditioning Engineers, 1978.

Amon, R.B., A.W. Lis, and J.M. Hanifin: Allergic Contact Dermatitis Caused by Idoxuridine. *Arch. Dermatol. 111:*1581-1584 (1975).

Anderson, D.C., P.A. Stoesz, and A.F. Kaufmann: Psittacosis Outbreak in Employees of a Turkey-Processing Plant. *Am. J. Epidemiol. 107:*140-148 (1978).

Anderson, R.E., L. Stein, M.D. Moss, and N.H. Gross: Potential Infectious Hazards of Common Bacteriological Techniques. *J. Bacteriol. 64:*473-481 (1952).

Anon.: Hazard Update — Risks from Centrifuges. *Health Devices 21(8):*290-291 (1992).

Anon.: *Occupational Diseases Acquired from Animals* (University of Michigan, School of Public Health, Continued Education Series No. 124). Ann Arbor, Mich.: University of Michigan, School of Public Health, 1964. p. 430.

Anon.: Review of Biosafety Guidelines. Biosafety Task Force, Parenteral Drug Association. *J. Parenteral Sci. & Tech. 43(6):*252-258 (1989).

Arbesman, C.E., R.B. Beede, and N.R. Rose: Sensitivity to Animals: A Case Report with Immunologic Studies. *J. Allergy 29:*129-183 (1958).

Ashdown, L.R.: Melioidosis and Safety in the Clinical Laboratory. *J. Hosp. Infect. 21(4):*301-306 (1992).

Bachner, P.: Teaching Safety Management Guidelines. *Am. J. Clin. Path. 96(4):*557 (1991).

Banazak, E.F., W.H. Thiede, and J.N. Fink: Hypersensitivity Pneumonitis Due to Contamination of an Air Conditioner. *New Eng. J. Med. 283(6):*271-276 (1970).

Bannerman, C.M., W.A. Black, and D.A. Black: A Technique for Bacteriological Sampling of Hair. *J. Clin. Pathol. 26(6):*448-449 (1973).

Barbeito, M.S., R.L. Alg, and A.G. Wedum: Infectious Bacterial Aerosol from Dropped Petri Dish Cultures. *Am. J. Med. Technol. 27:*318-322 (1961)

Barkley, W.E.: The Research Facility. In *Proceedings of the Workshop on Cancer Research Safety, September 26-29, 1977,* sponsored by National Cancer Institute, Office of Research Safety. Dulles Marriott Hotel, Dulles International Airport, Va., September 1977.

Barnes, R.: Industrial Dermatitis. *Med. J. Aust. 1:*850-854 (1970).

Batchelor, B.I., R.J. Brindle, G.F. Gilks, and J.B. Selkon: Biochemical Mis-identification of *Brucella melitensis* and Subsequent Laboratory-Acquired Infections. *J. Hosp. Infect. 22(2):*159-162 (1992).

Bauer, P.: Universal Precautions in OR Practice (I: Of Risks and Regulations). *Nursing Management 22(6):*56Q-56R, 56V, 56X (1991).

Behymer, D., and H.P. Riemann: *Coxiella Burnelii* Infection (Q Fever). *JAVMA 194(6):*764-767 (1989).

Biro, L., A.A. Fisher, and E. Price: Severe Burns Due to Residual Ethylene Oxide in Surgical Drapes. *Arch. Dermatol. 110:*924-925 (1974).

Brandt, R., G. Ponterius, and L. Yman: The Allergens of Cat Epithelia and Cat Serum. *Int. Arch. Allergy Appl. Immun. 45:*447-455 (1973).

Brewer, J.H. (ed.): *Lectures on Sterilization.* Durham, N.C.: Duke University Press, 1972.

Brinton, L.A., W.J. Blot, B.J. Stone, and J.F. Fraumeni, Jr.: A Death Certificate Analysis of Nasal Cancer Among Furniture Workers in North Carolina. *Cancer Res. 37:*3473-3474 (1977).

Broholm, K., A.M. Bottiger, H. Jernelius, M. Johansson, M.G. Grandien, and K. Solver: Ornithosis as a Nosocomial Infection. *Cand. J. Infect. Dis. 9:*263-267 (1977).

Brown, F., P. Talbot, and R. Burrows: Antigenic Differences Between Isolates of Swine Vesicular Virus and Their Relationship to Coxsackie B5 Virus. *Nature 245:*315-316 (1973).

Brown, J., J.L. Blue, R.E. Wooley, and D.W. Dressen: *Brucella canis* Infectivity Rates in Stray and Pet Dog Populations. *Am. J. Pub. Health 66:*889-892 (1976).

Brown, J.H., K.M. Cook, F.G. Ney, and T. Hatch: Influence of Particle Size Upon the Retention of Particulate Matter in the Human Being. *Am. J. Public Health 40:*450-458 (1950).

Bruins, S.C., and R.R. Tight: Laboratory-Acquired Gonococcal Conjunctivitis. *JAMA 241:*274 (1979).

Buesching, W.J., J.C. Neff, and H.M. Sharma: Infectious Hazards in the Clinical Laboratory: A Program to Protect Laboratory Personnel. *Clinics in Lab. Med. 9(2):*351-361 (1989).

Burgdorfer, W.: Q Fever. In *Diseases Transmitted from Animals to Man* (edited by W.T. Hubbert, W.F. McCulloch, and P.R. Schnurrenberger). Springfield, Ill.: Charles C. Thomas Publishers, 1975.

Burgdorfer, W.: Rocky Mountain Spotted Fever. In *Diseases Transmitted from Animals to Man* (edited by W.T. Hubbert, W.F. McCulloch, and P.R. Schnurrenberger). Springfield, Ill.: Charles C. Thomas Publishers, 1975.

Cate, L.T.: A Note on a Simple and Rapid Method of Bacteriological Sampling by Means of Agar Sausages. *J. Appl. Bacteriol 28(2):*221-223 (1965).

Centers for Disease Control and Prevention: *Brucellosis Surveillance Annual Summary.* Atlanta, Ga.: Centers for Disease Control and Prevention, 1976.

Centers for Disease Control and Prevention: *Classification of Etiologic Agents on the Basis of Hazard.* Atlanta, Ga.: Centers for Disease Control and Prevention, 1976.

Charpin, J: Occupational Asthma. In *Allergology* (edited by Y. Yamamura). Amsterdam: Excerpta Medica Foundation, 1974. pp. 120-122.

Chatigny, M.A.: Protection Against Infection in the Microbiological Laboratory: Devices and Procedures. *Adv. Appl. Microbiol. 3:*131-169 (1961).

Chatigny, M.A.: Sampling Airborne Microorganisms. In *Air Sampling Instruments for Evaluation of Atmospheric Contaminants,* 8th Edition. Cincinnati, Ohio: American Conference of Governmental Industrial Hygienists, 1995.

Chyrek, S., T. Karna, M. Gruszeka, D. Obrzut, and E. Kowal: Problems of Occupational Allergy in Health Service Workers. *Pol. Tyg. Lek. 31:*1393 (1976).

Cohen, B.J., and K.E. Brown: Laboratory Infection with Human Parvovirus B19. *J. Infect. 24(1):*113-1144 (1992).

Cohen, M.B., M.S. Zaleski, and R.P. Wenzel: AIDS-Related Safety Issues for the Cytology Laboratory. *Diagnostic Cytopathology 7(5):*543-545 (1991).

Cohen, R.C.: Desensitization of Hospital Staff to Streptomycin. *Tubercule 35:*142-144 (1954).

Colten, H.R., P.L. Polakoff, S.F. Weinstein, and D. Strieder: Immediate Hypersensitivity to Hog Trypsin from Industrial Exposure. *J. Allergy Clin. Immunol. 55:*130 (1975). [Abstract.]

Dance, D.A.: Melioidosis and Laboratory Safety. *J. Hosp. Infect. 22(4):*333-334 (1992). [Letter to the Editor.]

Dark, F.A., and G.J. Harper: Aerosol Sampling. In *Safety in Microbiology* (edited by D.A. Shapton and R.G. Board). New York: Academic Press, 1972.

Davies, R.J., and J. Pepys: Asthma Due to Inhaled Chemical Agents: The Macrolide Antibiotic Spiramycin. *Clin. Allergy 5:*99-107 (1975).

Davis, D.H.S., A.F. Hallett, and M. Isaacson: Plague. In *Diseases Transmitted from Animals to Man* (edited by W.T. Hubbert, W.F. McCulloch, and P.R. Schnurrenberger). Springfield, Ill.: Charles C. Thomas Publishers, 1975.

Decker, H.J., L.M. Buchanan, L.B. Hall, and K.R. Goddard: Air Filtration of Microbial Particles. *Am. J. Pub. Health 53:*1928-1988 (1963).

DeFeo, C.P.: Erythema Multiforme Bullosum Caused by 9-Bromofluorene. *Arch. Dermatol. 94:*545-551 (1966).

Diesch, S.L., and H.C. Ellinghausen: Leptospirosis. In *Diseases Transmitted from Animals to Man* (edited by W.T. Hubbert, W.F. McCulloch, and P.R. Schnurrenberger). Springfield, Ill.: Charles C. Thomas Publishers, 1975.

Dolovich, J., W. Shaikh, S. Tarlo, and F.E. Hargreave: Human Exposure and Sensitization to Airborne Papain. *Ann. Allergy 38:*94 (1977).

Druett, H.A., D.W. Henderson, L. Packman, and S. Peacock: Studies on Respiratory Infection (I. The Influence of Particle Size on Respiratory Infection with Anthrax Spores). *J. Hyg. 51:*359-371 (1953).

Dyer, R.E.: A Filter Passing Infectious Agent Isolated from Ticks in Montana. *Public Health Rep. U.S. 53:*2277-2282 (1938).

Evans, M.R., D.K. Henderson, and J.E. Bennett: Potential for Laboratory Exposures to Biohazardous Agents Found in Blood. *Am. J. Pub. Health 80(4):*423-427 (1990).

Favero, M.S., J.J. McDade, J.A. Robertsen, R.K. Hoffman, and R.W. Edwards: Microbiological Sampling of Surfaces. *J. Appl. Bacteriol. 31:*336-343 (1968).

Feinberg, S.M., and R.M. Watrous: Atopy to Simple Chemical Compounds, Sulfonechloramides. *J. Allergy 16:*209-220 (1945).

Fisher, A.A.: Allergic Contact Dermatitis in Animal Feed Handlers. *Cutis 16:*201-202 (1975).

Fisher, A.A.: Allergic Contact Sensitivity to Benzalkonium Chloride. Cutaneous, Ophthalmic, General Medical Implications. *Arch. Dermatol. 106:*169-171 (1972).

Fisher, A.A.: Hypoallergenic Surgical Gloves and Gloves for Special Situations. *Cutis 15:*797-806,811 (1975).

Fisher, A.A., F. Pascher, and N.B. Kanof: Allergic Contact Dermatitis Due to Ingredients of Vehicles. *Arch. Dermatol. 104:*286-290 (1971).

Fisher, J.J., and D.H. Walker: Invasive Pulmonary Aspergillosis Associated with Influenza. *JAVMA 241:*1493-1494 (1979).

Fox, J.G., and N.S. Lipman: Infections Transmitted by Large and Small Laboratory Animals. *Infect. Dis. Clin. North Am. 5(1):*131-163 (1991).

Frankland, A.E.: Rat Asthma in Laboratory Workers. In *Allergology* (edited by Y. Yamamura). Amsterdam: Excertpa Medica Foundation, 1974. p. 123.

Frommer, W., and P. Kramer: Safety Aspects in Biotechnology. Classifications and Safety Precautions for Handling of Biological Agents. *Arzneimittel-Forschung 40(7):*837-842 (1990).

Furcolow, M.L., W.G. Guntheroth, and M.J. Willis: The Frequency of Laboratory Infection with *Histoplasma capsulatum:* Their Clinical and X-Ray Characteristics. *J. Lab. Clin. Med. 40:*182-187 (1961).

Furuhashi, M., and T. Miyamae: Evaluation of the Commercial Bacterial Air Samples by the New Bacterial Aerosol Generator. *Bull. Tokyo Med. Dent. Univ. 28:*7-21 (1981).

Gandevia, B.: Occupational Asthma (Parts I and II). *Med. J. Aust. 2:*332-335 (1970).

Goldstein, L., and S. Johnson: OSHA Bloodborne Pathogens Standard. Implications for the Occupational Health Nurse. *AAOHNJ 39(4):*182-188 (1991).

Goodlow, R.S., and E.A. Leonard: Viability Infectivity of Microorganisms in Experimental Airborne Infections. *Bacteriol. Rev. 25:*182-187 (1961).

Graham, C.J., T. Yamauchi, and P. Rountree: Q Fever in Animal Laboratory Workers: An Outbreak and Its Investigation. *Am. J. Infect. Control 17(6):*345-348 (1989).

Gremillion, G.G.: The Use of Bacteria-Tight Cabinets in the Infectious Disease Laboratory. In *Proceedings of the 2nd Symposium on Gnotobiotic Technology.* South Bend, Ind.: University of Notre Dame Press, 1959.

Grist, N.R.: Hazards in the Clinical Pathology Laboratory. *Proc. R. Soc. Med. 66:*795-796 (1973). [Abstract.]

Grist, N.R.: Hepatitis in Clinical Laboratories: A Three-Year Survey. *J. Clin. Pathol. 28:*255-259 (1975).

Grist, N.R.: A Survey of Hepatitis in Laboratories. *J. Clin. Pathol. 26:*388 (1973).

Grist, N.R., and J.A. Emslie: Infections in British Clinical Laboratories. *J. Clin. Path. 42(7):*677-681 (1989).

Gross, H.T.: Erysipeloid: A Report of Thirteen Cases Among Veterinary Students at Kansas State College. *J. Kansas Med. Soc. 41:*329-332 (1940).

Hamadeh, G.N., B.W. Turner, W. Trible, Jr., B.J. Hoffman, and R.M. Anderson: Laboratory Outbreak of Q Fever. *J. Fam. Pract. 35(6):*683-685 (1992).

Hambleton, P., and G. Dedonato: Protecting Researchers from Instrument Biohazards. *Biotechniques 13(3):*450-453 (1992).

Hambraeus, A., and G. Laurell: Infections in a Burn Unit. *Contribut. Microbiol. Immunol. 1:*459-468 (1973).

Hamilton, A., and H.L. Hardy: *Industrial Toxicology, 3rd Ed.* Acton, Mass.: Publishing Sciences Group, Inc., 1974.

Hanel, E., Jr., and R.L. Alg: Biological Hazards of Common Laboratory Procedures (II. The Hypodermic Syringe and Needle). *Am. J. Med. Technol. 21:*343-346 (1955).

Hanson, P., S.E. Sulkin, E.L. Buescher, W. McD. Hammon, R.W. McKinney, and T.H. Work: Arbovirus Infection of Laboratory Workers. *Science 158:*1283-1286 (1967).

Hanson, R.P.: Paramyxovirus Infections. In *Diseases Transmitted from Animals to Man* (edited by W.T. Hubbert, W.F. McCulloch, and P.R. Schnurrenberger). Springfield, Ill.: Charles C. Thomas Publishers, 1975.

Harrington, J.M., and H.S. Shannon: Survey of Safety and Health Care in British Medical Laboratories. *Brit. Med. J. 1:*626-628 (1977).

Hellman, A.: *Biohazard Control and Containment in Oncogenic Virus Research.* Bethesda, Md.: U.S. Department of Health, Education, and Welfare, National Institutes of Health, 1969.

Hellman, A., M.N. Oxman, and R. Pollack (eds): *Biohazards in Biological Research.* Cold Spring Harbor, N.Y.: Cold Spring Harbor Laboratory, 1973.

Hendrick, D.S., and D.J. Lane: Occupational Formalin Asthma. *Brit. J. Ind. Med. 34:*11-18 (1977).

Hendricks, S.L., and M.E. Meyer: Brucellosis. In *Diseases Transmitted from Animals to Man* (edited by W.T. Hubbert, W.F. McCulloch, and P.R. Schnurrenberger). Springfield, Ill.: Charles C. Thomas Publishers, 1975.

Huddleson, I.F., and M. Munger: A Study of an Epidemic of Brucellosis Due to *Brucella melitensis. Am. J. Public Health 30:*944-945 (1940).

Jemski, J.V.: Maintenance of Monkeys Experimentally Infected with Organisms Pathogenic for Man. *Proc. Anim. Care Panel 12:*89-98 (1962).

Jemski, J.V., and G.B. Phillips: Microbiological Safety Equipment. *Lab. Anim. Care 13:*2-12 (1963).

Jones, A.W.: *Introduction to Parasitology.* Reading, Mass.: Addison-Wesley Publishing Co., 1967.

Jordon, W.P., Jr., M. Dahl, and H.L. Albert: Contact Dermatitis from Gluteraldehyde. *Arch. Dermatol. 105:*94-95 (1972).

Kahn, G.: Depigmentation Caused by Phenolic Detergent Germicides. *Arch. Dermtol. 102:*177-187 (1970).

Kanof, N.B., and E. Biondi: Routine Screening Patch Test Results. *Cutis 18:*668-669 (1976).

Kimondollo, P.M.: Guidelines for Developing a Dental Laboratory Infection-Control Protocol. *Int. J. Prosthodontics 5(5):*452-456 (1992).

Kirchheimer, W.F., J.V. Jemski, and G.B. Phillips: Cross-Infection Among Experimental Animals by Organisms Infectious for Man. *Proc. Anim. Care Panel 11:*83-92 (1961).

Kisskalt, K: Laboratory Infections with Typhoid Bacilli. *Zeitschrift fur Hygiene and Infektions Krankheiten 80:*145-162 (1915).

Kissling, R.E.: Herpesviruses. In *Diseases Transmitted from Animals to Man* (edited by W.T. Hubbert, W.F. McCulloch, and P.R. Schnurrenberger). Springfield, Ill.: Charles C. Thomas Publishers, 1975.

Kissling, R.E.: Marburg Virus. In *Diseases Transmitted from Animals to Man* (edited by W.T. Hubbert, W.F. McCulloch, and P.R. Schnurrenberger). Springfield, Ill.: Charles C. Thomas Publishers, 1975.

Kruse, R.H., W.H. Puckett, and J.H. Richardson: Biological Safety Cabinetry. *Clin. Microbiology Rev. 4(2):*207-241 (1991).

Lairmore, M.D., J.E. Kaplan, M.D. Daniel, N.W. Lerche, P.L. Nara, H.M. McClure, J.W. McVicar, R.W. McKinney, M. Hendry, P. Gerone, et al.: Guidelines for the Prevention of Simian Immunodeficiency Virus Infection in Laboratory Workers and Animal Handlers. *J. Med. Primatology 18(3-4):*167-174 (1989).

Larson, E.L., M.S. Strom, and C.A. Evans: Analysis of Three Variables in Sampling Solutions Used to Assay Bacteria of Hands: Type of Solution, Use of Antiseptic Neutralizers, and Solution Temperature. *J. Clin. Microbiol. 12(3):*355-360 (1980).

Lass, N., and H. Arion: Medico-Legal Aspects of Occupational Asthma. In *Allergology* (edited by Y. Yamamura). Amsterdam: Excerpta Medica Foundation, 1974. pp. 133-138.

Lesko, J.: Biohazard in Microbiology, Virology and in Work with Cell Cultures. *Sbornik Vedeckych Praci Lekarske Fakulty Karlovy Univerzity V Hradci Kralove. 33(2):*89-94 (1990).

Levene, G.M., and A.F.D. Withers: Anaphylaxis to Streptomycin and Hyposensitization (Parasensitization). *Trans. Rep. St. John's Hospital Derm. Soc. 55:*184 (1969).

Liberman, D.F., and R. Fink: Containment Considerations for the Biotechnology Industry. *State of the Art Reviews: Occupational Medicine 6(2):*271-283 (1991).

Little, P.J., and K.L. Lynn: Neomycin Toxicity. *New Zealand J. Med. 81:*445 (1975). [Letter to the Editor.]

Litton Bionetics, Inc.: *Packages for Shipment of Etiologic Agents, Tested for Compliance with the Environment and Test Conditions Prescribed by the Department of Transportation, Environmental and Industrial Safety and Health.* Frederick, Md.: Litton Bionetics, Inc., 1974.

Meyer, K.F., and B. Eddie: Laboratory Infections Due to *Brucell. J. Infect. Dis. 68:*24-32 (1941).

Morris, E.J.: A Survey of Safety Precautions in the Microbiological Laboratory. *J. Med. Lab. Technol. 17:*70-81 (1960).

Most, H.: *Plasmodium cynomolgi* Malaria: Accidental Human Infection. *Am. J. Trop. Med. Hyg. 22:*157-158 (1973).

Nater, J.P.: Allergic Reactions Due to Chloroacetamide. *Contact Derm. Newsletter 8:*176 (1970).

National Sanitation Foundation: *NSF Standard No. 49 for Class II (Laminar Flow) Biohazard Cabinetry.* Ann Arbor, Mich.: National Sanitation Foundation, 1976.

Nava, C.: Allergic Manifestations Due to d1-Cycloserine (Oxamycin). *Med. Lav. 62:*335-344 (1971).

Neuman, I., and I. Lutsky: Laboratory Animal Dander Allergy (II. Clinical Studies and the Potential Protective Effect of Disodium Chromoglycate). *Ann. Allergy 36:*23-29 (1976).

Nguyen, C., and R.G. Lalonde: Risk of Occupational Exposure to *Herpesvirus simiae* (B virus) in Quebec. *Canadian Med. Assoc. J. 143(11):*1203-1206 (1990).

Niskanen, A., and M.S. Pohja: Comparative Studies on the Sampling and Investigation of Microbial Contamination of Surfaces by the Contact Plate and Swab Methods. *J. Appl. Bact. 42:*53-63 (1977).

Odom, R.B., and H.I. Maibach: Contact Urticaria: A Different Contact Dermatitis. *Cutis 18:*672-676 (1976).

Ohman, J.L.: Allergy in Man Caused by Exposure to Mammals. *JAVMA 172:*1403-1406 (1978).

Olsen, P.F.: Tularemia. In *Diseases Transmitted from Animals to Man* (edited by W.T. Hubbert, W.F. McCulloch, and P.R. Schnurrenberger). Springfield, Ill.: Charles C. Thomas Publishers, 1975.

Osborne, R.W., and T.A. Durkin: Continued Successful Operation of Open-Fronted Microbiological Safety Cabinets in a Force-Ventilated Laboratory. *J. Appl. Bact. 71(5):*434-438 (1991).

Parker, S.L., and R.E. Holliman: Toxoplasmosis and Laboratory Workers: A Case-Control Assessment of Risk. *Med. Lab. Sci. 49(2):*103-106 (1992).

Patterson, R.: The Problem of Allergy to Laboratory Animals. *Lab. Animal Care 14:*466-469 (1964).

Pegum, J.S., and F.A. Medhurst: Contact Dermatitis from Penetration of Rubber Gloves by Acrylic Monomer. *Brit. Med. J. 2:*141-143 (1971).

Pepys, J., and R.J. Davies: Occupational Asthma. In *Allergy: Principles and Practice* (edited by Middleton, Ellis, and Reed). St. Louis: Mosby, 1978.

Pepys, J., C.A.C. Pickering, and H.W.G. Loudon: Asthma Due to Inhaled Chemical Agents — Piperazine Hydrochloride. *Clin. Allergy 2:*189-196 (1972).

Phillips, G.B.: Causal Factors in Microbiological Laboratory Accidents and Infections (Misc. Publication 2). Fort Detrick, Md.: U.S. Army Biological Laboratories, 1965. p. 251.

Phillips, G.B.: Control of Microbiological Hazards in the Laboratory. *Am. Ind. Hyg. Assoc. J. 30:*170-176 (March-April 1969).

Phillips, G.B: *Laboratory Infections Bibliography.* Research Triangle Park, N.C.: Becton, Dickinson and Company, 1975.

Phillips, G.B.: Microbiological Hazards in the Laboratory (I. Control). *J. Chem. Educ. 42:*A43-A48 (1965).

Phillips, G.B.: Microbiological Hazards in the Laboratory (II. Prevention). *J. Chem. Educ. 42:*A117-A130 (1965).

Phillips, G.B.: *Microbiological Safety in U.S. and Foreign Laboratories* (Technical Report BL 35). Fort Detrick, Md.: U.S. Army Chemical Corps, Biological Laboratories, 1961.

Phillips, G.B., and S.P. Baley: Hazards of Mouth Pipetting. *Am. J. Med. Technol. 32:*127-129 (1966).

Phillips, G.B., and J.V. Jemski: Biological Safety in the Animal Laboratory. *Lab. Animal Care 13:*13-20 (1963).

Phillips, G.B., and J.V. Jemski: *Microbiological Safety Bibliography* (Misc. Publication 6). Fort Detrick, Md.: U.S. Army Biological Laboratories, 1965.

Phillips, G.B., and W.S. Miller (eds.): *Industrial Sterilization.* Durham, N.C.: Duke University Press, 1972.

Phillips, G.B., and M. Reitman: Biological Hazards of Common Laboratory Procedures (IV. The Inoculating Loop). *Am. J. Med. Technol. 22:*16-17 (1956).

Phillips, G.B., M. Reitman, C.L. Mullican, and G.D. Gardner: Applications of Germicidal Ultraviolet in Infectious Disease Laboratories (III. The Use of Ultraviolet Barriers on Animal Cage Racks). *Proc. Anim. Care Panel 7:*235-244 (1957).

Phillips, G.B., and R.S. Runkle: *Biomedical Applications of Laminar Airflow.* Cleveland, Ohio: CRC Press, Div. of Chemical Rubber Company, 1973.

Phillips, G.B., and R.S. Runkle: Laboratory Design for Microbiological Safety. *App. Microbiol. 15:*378-389 (1967).

Pike, R.M., and S.E. Sulkin: Occupational Hazards in Microbiology. *Sci. Month. 75:*222-228 (1952).

Pike, R.M., S.E. Sulkin, and M.L. Schulze: Continuing Importance of Laboratory-Acquired Infections. *Am. J. Public Health 55:*190-199 (1965).

Pittman, B., E.B. Shaw, Jr., and W.B. Cherry: Isolation of *Francisella tularensis* from Infected Frozen Human Blood. *J. Clin. Microbiol. 5:*621-624 (1977).

Powell, K.E., A. Taylor, B.J. Phillips, D.L. Blakey, S.D. Campbell, L. Kaufman, and W. Kaplan: Cutaneous Sporotonicous in Forestry Workers. *JAVMA 240:*232-235.

Press, E., J.A. Goojins, H. Poareo, and K. Jones: Health Hazards to Timber and Forestry Workers from the Douglas Fir Tussock Moth. *Arch. Env. Health 32:*206-210 (1977).

Rajka, G.: Ten Cases of Occupational Hypersensitivity to Laboratory Animals. *Acta. Allergol. 16:*168-176 (1964).

Reinhardt, D.J., W. Nabors, C. Kennedy, and B. Malecka-Griggs: Limulus Amoebocyte Lysate and Direct Sampling Methods for Surveillance of Operating Nebulizers. *Appl. Environ. Microbiol. 42(5):*850-855 (1981).

Reitman, M., and G.B. Phillips: Biological Hazards of Common Laboratory Procedures (I. The Pipette). *Am. J. Med. Technol. 21:*338-342 (1955).

Reitman, M., and G.B. Phillips: Biological Hazards of Common Laboratory Procedures (III. The Centrifuge). *Am. J. Med. Technol. 22:*14-16 (1955).

Reitman, M., M.S. Frank, Sr., R. Alg, and A.G. Wedum: Infectious Hazards of the High Speed Blender and Their Elimination by a New Design. *Appl. Microbiol. 1:*14-17 (1953).

Reitman, M., M.L. Moss, J.B. Harstad, R.L. Alg, and N.H. Gross: Potential Infectious Hazards of Laboratory Techniques (I. Lyophilization). *J. Bacteriol. 68:*541-544 (1954).

Reitman, M., M.L. Moss, J.B. Harstad, R.L. Alg, and N.H. Gross: Potential Infectious Hazards of Laboratory Techniques. (II. The Handling of Lyophilized Cultures). *J. Bacteriol. 68:*545-548 (1954).

Reitman, M., R.L. Alg, W.S. Miller, and N.H. Gross: Potential Infectious Hazards of Laboratory Techniques (III. Viral Techniques). *J. Bacteriol. 68:*549-554 (1954).

Ridgway, G.L.: Preventing Infection in Laboratories. *Brit. Med. J. 304(6819):*66-67 (1992).

Robbins, F.C., and R. Rustigion: Q Fever in the Mediterranean Area: Report of Its Occurrence in Allied Troops (II. A Laboratory Outbreak). *Am. J. Hyg. 44:*64-71 (1946).

Roed-Peterson, J., and T. Menne: Allergic Contact Dermatitis and Lichen Planus from Black and White Photographic Developing. *Cutis 18:*699-705 (1976).

Rudziki, E.: Cross Reactions in Occupational Contact Dermatitis (I. Aromatic Amines). *Berufsdermatosen 25:*236-245 (1977).

Ryan, K.J., and S.F. Mihalyi: Evaluation of a Simple Device for Bacteriological Sampling of Respirator-Generated Aerosols. *J. Clin. Microbiol. 5(2):*178-183 (1977).

Sabin, A.B., and A.M. Wright: Acute Ascending Myelitis Following Monkey Bite, with Isolation of Virus Capable of Reproducing Disease. *J. Exp. Med. 59:*115-136 (1934).

Schick, G.: Microsporum Dermatomycosis of Laboratory Origin. *Berufsdermatosen 16:*34-42 (1970).

Schrader, S.M.: Safety Guidelines for the Andrology Laboratory. *Fertility & Sterility 51(3):*387-389 (1989).

Schultz, K.H., E. Schopf, and O. Wex: Occupational Eczema Caused by Ampicillin. *Berufsdermatosen 18:*132 (1970).

Seaton, A.: Occupational Asthma. In *Occupational Lung Diseases* (edited by K.C. Morgan and A. Seaton). Philadelphia: W.B. Saunders Co., 1975. p. 251.

Selby, L.A.: Blastomycosis. In *Diseases Transmitted from Animals to Man* (edited by W.T. Hubbert, W.F. McCulloch, and P.R. Schnurrenberger). Springfield, Ill.: Charles C. Thomas Publishers, 1975.

Selby, L.A.: Coccidioidomycosis. In *Diseases Transmitted from Animals to Man* (edited by W.T. Hubbert, W.F. McCulloch, and P.R. Schnurrenberger). Springfield, Ill.: Charles C. Thomas Publishers, 1975.

Selby, L.A.: Histoplasmosis. In *Diseases Transmitted from Animals to Man* (edited by W.T. Hubbert, W.F. McCulloch, and P.R. Schnurrenberger). Springfield, Ill.: Charles C. Thomas Publishers, 1975.

Sharma, V.K., B. Kumar, B.D. Radorta, and S. Kaur: Cutaneous Inoculation Tuberculosis in Laboratory Personnel. *Int. J. Dermatology 29(4):*293-294 (1990).

Shaw, C.M., J.A. Smith, M.E. McBride, and W.C. Duncan: An Evaluation of Techniques for Sampling Skin Flora. *J. Invest. Dermatol. 54(2):*160-162 (1970).

Sikes, R.K., Sr.: Rabies. In *Diseases Transmitted from Animals to Man* (edited by W.T. Hubbert, W.F. McCulloch, and P.R. Schnurrenberger). Springfield, Ill.: Charles C. Thomas Publishers, 1975.

Staszkiewicz, J., C.M. Lewis, J. Colville, M. Zervow, and J. Band: Outbreak of *Brucella Melitensis* Among Microbiology Laboratory Workers in a Community Hospital. *J. Clin. Microbiology 29(2):*287-290 (1991).

Stern, E.L., J.W. Johnson, D. Vesley, M.M. Halbert, L.E. Williams, and P. Blume: Aerosol Production Associated with Clinical Laboratory Procedures. *Am. J. Clin. Pathol. 62:*591-600 (1974).

Storrs, F.J.: Para-chloro-meta-xylenol Allergic Contact Dermatitis in Seven Individuals. *Contact Derm. 1:*211 (1975).

Sulkin, S.E.: Laboratory-Acquired Infections. *Bact. Rev. 25:*203-209 (1961).

Sulkin, S.E., and R.M. Pike: Laboratory-Acquired Infections. *J. Am. Med. Assoc. 147:*1740-1745 (1951).

Sulkin, S.E., and R.M. Pike: Survey of Laboratory-Acquired Infections. *Am. J. Public Health 41:*769-781 (1951).

Sulkin, S.E., and R.M. Pike: Viral Infections Contracted in the Laboratory. *New Eng. J. Med. 241:*205-213 (1949).

Sulkin, S.E., E.R. Long, R.M. Pike, M.M. Siegel, C.E. Smith, and A.G. Wedum: Laboratory Infections and Accidents. In *Diagnostic Procedures and Reagents, 4th Ed.* (edited by A.H. Harrison and M.B. Coleman). New York: Am. Pub. Health Assoc., Inc., 1963. pp. 89-104.

Sullivan, J.F., J.R. Songer, and I.E. Estrem: Laboratory-Acquired Infections at the National Animal Disease Center, 1960-1976. *Health Lab. Sci. 15:*58-64 (1977).

Tamminga, S.K., and E.H. Kampelmacher: Comparison of Agar Sausage, Alginate Swab and Adhesive Tape Methods for Sampling Flat Surfaces Contaminated with Bacteria. *Abl. Bakt. Hyg., Abt. Orig. B. 165:*423-434 (1977).

Tesh, R.B., and K.M. Johnson: Vesicular Stomatitis. In *Diseases Transmitted from Animals to Man* (edited by W.T. Hubbert, W.F. McCulloch, and P.R. Schnurrenberger). Springfield, Ill.: Charles C. Thomas Publishers, 1975.

Tousch, B.: Cutaneomucosal Accidents with Sulfonamides. *Rev. Stomtol. (Paris) 77:*721-726 (1971).

U.S. Department of Health, Education and Welfare: *Occupational Diseases: A Guide to Their Recognition* (DHEW No. 77-181). Washington, D.C.: U.S. Government Printing Office, 1977.

Van Arsdel, P.O.: Adverse Drug Reactions. In *Allergy, Principles and Practice* (edited by Middleton, Reed, and Ellis). St. Louis: Mosby, 1978.

Vetter, T.R., and B. Kuzma: Secondary Sharps Container. *Anesthesiology 78(3):*611 (1993).

Voss, H.E.: Clinical Detection of the Potential Allergic Reaction to Penicillin by Immunologic Tests. *JAMA 196:*679-683 (1966).

Wedum, A.G.: Control of Laboratory Airborne Infection. *Bacteriol. Rev. 25:*210-216 (1961).

Wedum, A.G.: "History of Microbiological Safety." Paper presented at the 18th Biological Safety Conference, Lexington, Ky., 1975.

Wedum, A.G.: Laboratory Safety in Research with Infectious Aerosols. *Public Health Report 78:*619-633 (1964).

Wedum, A.G., W.E. Barkley, and A. Hellman: Handling of Infectious Agents. *JAVMA 161(11):*1557-1567 (1972).

Wedum, A.G., E. Hanel, G.B. Phillips, and O.T. Miller: Laboratory Design for Study of Infectious Diseases. *Am. J. Pub. Health 46:*1102-1113 (1956).

Wedum, A.G., and R.H. Kruse: *Assessment of Risk of Human Infection in the Microbiological Laboratory.* Fort Detrick, Md.: U.S. Department of the Army, 1966.

West, D.L., D.R. Twardzik, R.W. McKinney, W.E. Barkeley, and A. Hellman: Identification, Analysis and Control of Biohazards in Viral Cancer Research. In *Laboratory Safety* (edited by A.A. Fuscaldo, B.J. Erlick, and B. Hindman). New York: Academic Press, 1980. pp. 167-223.

Whitehead, W.J., J.R. Beakley, V.I. Dugan, I.W. Highes, M.E. Morris, and J.J. McDade: Vacuum Probes: New Approach to Microbiological Sampling of Surfaces. *Appl. Microbiol. 17:*164-168 (1969).

Williams, L.P., and B.C. Hobbs: Enterobacteriaceae Infections. In *Diseases Transmitted from Animals to Man* (edited by W.T. Hubbert, W.F. McCulloch, and P.R. Schnurrenberger). Springfield, Ill.: Charles C. Thomas Publishers, 1975.

Wilson, J.A.: Hamster-Hair Hypersensitivity in Adults of Low Atopic Status. *Brit. Med. J. 4:*341 (1971).

Wolff, M.: Eure Einfache und Dauerhafte Saugipette sum Gebrauch bei Mikroskopischen Arbeiten Zentralbe. [Our Simple and Durable Suction Pipette for Use With Microscopic Investigations.] *Bakteriol. 46:*648-651 (1908). [German.]

Woo, J.H., J.Y. Cho, Y.S. Kin, D.H. Choi, N.M. Lee, K.W. Choe, and W.H. Chang: A Case of Laboratory-Acquired Murine Typhus. *Korean J. Internal Med. 5(2):*118-122 (1990).

Wood, R.L.: Erysipelothrix Infection. In *Diseases Transmitted from Animals to Man* (edited by W.T. Hubbert, W.F. McCulloch, and P.R. Schnurrenberger). Springfield, Ill.: Charles C. Thomas Publishers, 1975.

Wright, G.G.: Anthrax. In *Diseases Transmitted from Animals to Man* (edited by W.T. Hubbert, W.F. McCulloch, and P.R. Schnurrenberger). Springfield, Ill.: Charles C. Thomas Publishers, 1975.

Ziegler, V., W. Bucholz, E. Suss, and O. Petter: Epidemiologische Studie Professionaller Kontaktekzeme in Gesundheidtswesen. [Epidemiological Study of Occupational Contact Eczema in Health Concerns.] *Dtsch. Gesundheidtsw. 27:*2195 (1972). [German.]

ADDITIONAL REFERENCES FOR BIOAEROSOL SAMPLING:

Andersen, A.A.: New Sampler for the Collection, Sizing, and Enumeration of Viable Airborne Particles. *J. Bacteriol. 76:*471-484 (1958).

Anderson Samplers, Inc.: *Model 10-880 Single Stage Bioaerosol Sampler.* Atlanta, Ga.: Anderson Samplers, Inc.

Anderson Samplers, Inc.: *Sampling for Airborne Microorganisms (Anderson Microbial Air Sampler).* Atlanta, Ga.: Anderson Samplers, Inc.

Blomquist, G., G. Ström, and L.-H. Strömquist: Sampling of High Concentrations of Airborne Fungi. *Scand. J. Work. Environ. Hlth 10:*109-113 (1984).

Brachman, P.S., R. Ehrlich, H.F. Eichenwald, V.J. Gabelli, T.W. Kethley, S.H. Madin, J.R. Maltman, G. Middlebrook, J.D. Morton, I.H. Silver, and E.K. Wolfe: Standard Sampler for Assay of Airborne Microorganisms. *Science:1295* (June 1964).

Burge, H.A., and W.R. Solomon: Sampling and Analysis of Biological Aerosols. *Atmospheric Environment 21(2):*451-456 (1987).

Burge, H.A., J.R. Boise, J.A. Rutherford, and W.R. Solomon: Comparative Recoveries of Airborne Fungus Spores by Viable and Non-Viable Modes of Volumetric Collection. *Mycopathologia 61(1):*27-33 (1977).

Burge, H.A., M. Chatigny, J. Feeley, K. Kreiss, P. Morey, J. Otten, and K. Peterson: Bioaerosols: Guidelines for Assessment and Sampling of Saprophytic Bioaerosols in the Indoor Environment. *Appl. Ind. Hyg. 2(5):*R10-R16 (1987).

Donham, K.J., L.J. Scallon, W. Popendorf, M.W. Treuhaft, and R.C. Roberts: Characterization of Dusts Collected from Swine Confinement Buildings. *Am. Ind. Hyg. Assoc. J. 47:*404-410 (1986).

Dutkiewicz, J.: Exposure to Dust and Bacteria in Agriculture Environmental Studies. *Appl. Environ. Microbiol. 33:*250-259 (1978).

Eduard, W., and O. Aalen: The Effect of Aggregation on the Counting Precision of Mould Spores on Filters. *Ann. Occup. Hyg. 32(4):*471-479 (1988).

Eickhoff, T.C., V.W. Greene, L.H. Herman, L.J. Hart, and G.F. Mallison: "Role of Environmental Sampling." In *Proceedings of the International Conference on Nosocomial Infections,* American Hospital Association, 1971. pp. 265-271.

Favero, M.S., and J.R. Puleo: Techniques Used for Sampling Airborne Microorganisms Associated with Industrial Clean Rooms and Spacecraft Assembly Areas. *Ann. New York Acad. Sci.:*241-253 (1980).

Hirst, J.M.: An Automatic Volumetric Spore Trap. *Ann. Appl. Biol. 39:*257 (1952).

Hobbie, J.E., R.J. Daley, and S. Jasper: Use of Nucleopore Filters for Counting Bacteria by Fluorescence Microscopy. *Appl. and Environ. Microbiol. 33(5):*1225-1228 (1977).

Holt, G.L.: "Seasonal Indoor/Outdoor Fungi Ratios and Indoor Bacteria Levels in Noncompliant Office Buildings." In *Proceedings of the Fifth International Conference on Indoor Air Quality and Climate, Toronto, Canada, July 29-August 3, 1990, Vol. 2.* pp. 33-38.

Jacobs, R.R.: Airborne Endotoxins: An Association with Occupational Lung Disease. *Appl. Ind. Hyg. 4:*50-55 (1989).

Jones, W., K. Morring, S. Olenchock, T. Williams, and J. Hickey: Environmental Study of Poultry Confinement Buildings. *Am. Ind. Hyg. Assoc. J. 45:*760-766 (1984).

Karlsson, K., and P. Malmberg: Characterization of Exposure to Molds and Actinomycetes in Agricultural Dusts by Scanning Electron Microscopy, Fluorescence Microscopy and the Culture Method. *Scand. J. Work. Environ. Hlth. 15:*353-359 (1989).

Lacey, J., and B. Crook: Review: Fungal and Actinomycete Spores as Pollutants of the Workplace and Occupational Allergens. *Ann. Occup. Hyg. 32(4):*515-533 (1988).

Lacey, J., and J. Dutkiewicz: Isolation of Actinomycetes and Fungi from Mouldy Hay Using a Sedimentation Chamber. *J. Appl. Bacterio. 41:*315-319 (1976).

Lacey, J., and J. Dutkiewicz: Methods for Examining and Microflora of Mouldy Hay. *J. Appl. Bacterio. 41:*13-27 (1976).

Lorincz, A.E.: Rapid Fluorescence Technique for the Detection of Toxic Pulmonary Microorganisms, e.g. Legionella Pneumophila. In *Manual of Procedures for Clinical and Analytical Toxicology* (edited by F. William Sunderman). Institute for Clinical Sciences, Inc., 1987. pp. 129-131.

Macher, J.M.: Positive-Hole Correction of Multiple-Jet Impactors for Collecting Viable Microorganisms. *Am. Ind. Hyg. Assoc. J. 50:*561-568 (1989).

Macher, J.M., and M.W. First: Personal Air Samplers for Measuring Occupational Exposures to Biological Hazards. *Am. Ind. Hyg. Assoc. J. 45:*76-83 (1984).

Martinez, K.F., J.W. Sheehy, J.H. Jones, and L.B. Cusick: Microbial Containment in Conventional Fermentation Processes. *Appl. Ind. Hyg. 3:*177-181 (1988).

May, K.R.: The Cascade Impactor: An Instrument for Sampling Coarse Aerosols. *J. Sci. Instr. 22:*187 (1945).

McGarrity, G.J., L.L. Coriell, R.W. Schaedler, R.J. Mandle, and A.E. Greene: Studies on Airborne Infection in Animal Care Laboratory. *Developments in Industrial Microbiology II:*58-64 (1970).

Milton, D.K., R.J. Gere, H.A. Feldman, and I.A. Greaves: Endotoxin Measurement: Aerosol Sampling and Application of a New Limulus Method. *Am. Ind. Assoc. J. 51:*331-337 (1990).

Morring, K.L., W.G. Sorenson, and M.D. Attfield: Sampling for Airborne Fungi: A Statistical Comparison of Media. *Am. Ind. Hyg. Assoc. J. 44(9):*662-664 (1983).

Nilsson, C.: *Dust Investigations in Pig Houses: Report 25.* Lund, Sweden: Dept. of Farm Buildings, Swedish Agricultural University, 1982.

Nordic Council of Ministers.: *Harmonization of Sampling and Analysis of Mould Spores.* Copenhagen: Nordic Council of Ministers, 1988.

Palmgren, U., G. Stroem, G. Blomquist, and P. Malmberg: Collection of Airborne Micro-organisms on Nuclepore Filters. Estimation and Analysis — CAMNEA Method. *J. Appl. Bacteriol.* *61:*401-406 (1986).

Pasanen, A.-L., P. Kalliokoski, P. Pasanen, T. Salmi, and An. Tossavainen: Fungi Carried from Farmers' Work into Farm Homes. *Am. Ind. Hyg. Assoc. J. 50(12):*631-633 (1989).

Popendorf, W.: Report on Agents. *Am. J. Indus. Med. 10:*251-259 (1986).

Reque, P.G., and A.E. Lorincz: Supravital Microscopic Fluorescent Technique for the Detection of Tinea Capitis. *Cutis 42:*111-114 (August 1988).

Runkle, R.S., and G.B. Phillips (eds.): *Biological Monitoring of the Environment — Microbial Contamination Control Facilities.* New York: Van Nostrand Reinhold Company, 1969. pp. 157-158.

Rylander, R., and J. Vesterlund: Airborne Endotoxins in Various Occupational Environments. *Prog. Clin. Biol. Res. 93:*399-409 (1982).

Smid, T., E. Schokkin, J.S.M. Boleij, and D. Heekerik: Enumeration of Viable Fungi in Occupational Environments: A Comparison of Samplers and Media. *Am. Ind. Hyg. Assoc. J. 50(5):*235-239 (1989).

Society for General Microbiology: *Seventeenth Symposium: Airborne Microbes.* London: Cambridge University Press, 1967. pp. 60-101.

Zimmerman, N.J., P.C. Reist, and A.G. Turner: Comparison of Two Biological Aerosol Sampling Methods. *Appl. Environ. Microb. 53:*99-104 (1987).

Appendix II

Biosafety Level Criteria for Infectious Agents *

The essential elements of the four biosafety levels for activities involving infectious agents are summarized in Table I below. The levels are designated in ascending order, by degree of protection provided to personnel, the environment, and the community.

Biosafety Level 1 (BSL1) is suitable for work involving agents of no known or of minimal potential hazard to laboratory personnel and the environment. The laboratory is not separated from the general traffic patterns in the building. Work generally is conducted on open bench tops. Special containment equipment is not required or generally used. Laboratory personnel have specific training in the procedures conducted in the laboratory and are supervised by a scientist with general training in microbiology or a related science.

The following standard and special practices, safety equipment, and facilities apply to agents assigned to BSL1:

A. *Standard Microbiological Practices*

1. Access to the laboratory is limited or restricted at the discretion of the laboratory director when experiments are in progress.
2. Work surfaces are decontaminated once a day and after any spill of viable material.
3. All contaminated liquid or solid wastes are decontaminated before disposal.
4. Mechanical pipetting devices are used; mouth pipetting is prohibited.

Table I. Summary of Recommended Biosafety Levels for Infectious Diseases

Biosafety Level	Practices and Techniques	Safety Equipment	Facilities
1	Standard microbiological practices	None: primary containment by adherence to standard laboratory practices during open bench operations.	Basic
2	Level 1 practices, plus: laboratory coats; decontamination of all infectious wastes; limited access; protective gloves and biohazard warning signs as indicated.	Partial containment equipment (i.e., Class I or II biological safety cabinets) used to conduct mechanical manipulative procedures that might increase the risk of exposure to personnel.	Basic
3	Level 2 practices, plus: special laboratory clothing; controlled access.	Partial containment equipment used for all manipulations of infectious material.	Containment
4	Level 3 practices, plus: entrance through clothes-change room where street clothing is removed and laboratory clothing is put on; shower on exit; all wastes are decontaminated on exit from the facility.	Maximum containment equipment (i.e., Class III biological safety cabinet or partial containment equipment in combination with full-body, air-supplied, positive-pressure personnel suit) used for all procedures and activities.	Maximum Containment

* Adapted from *Biosafety in Microbiological and Biomedical Laboratories*, 3rd Ed., USDHHS, USPHS, CDC, NIH, May 1993.

5. Eating, drinking, smoking, and applying cosmetics are not permitted in the work area. Food may be stored in cabinets or refrigerators designated and used for this purpose only. Food storage cabinets or refrigerators should be located outside of the work area.
6. Persons wash their hands after they handle viable materials and animals and before leaving the laboratory.
7. All procedures are performed carefully to minimize the creation of aerosols.
8. It is recommended that laboratory coats, gowns, or uniforms be worn to prevent contamination or soiling of street clothes.

B. *Special Practices*

1. Contaminated materials that are to be decontaminated at a site away from the laboratory are placed in a durable, leakproof container which is closed before being removed from the laboratory.
2. An insect and rodent control program is in effect.

C. *Containment Equipment*

Special containment equipment is generally not required for manipulations of agents assigned to BSL1.

D. *Laboratory Facilities*

1. The laboratory is designed so it can be cleaned easily.
2. Bench tops are impervious to water and resistant to acids, alkalis, organic solvents and moderate heat.
3. Laboratory furniture is sturdy. Spaces between benches, cabinets, and equipment are accessible for cleaning.
4. Each laboratory contains a sink for handwashing.
5. If the laboratory has windows that open, they are fitted with fly screens.

Biosafety Level 2 (BSL2) is similar to BSL1 and is suitable for work involving agents of moderate potential hazard to personnel and the environment. It differs in that 1) laboratory personnel have specific training in handling pathogenic agents and are directed by competent scientists; 2) access to the laboratory is limited when work is being conducted; and 3) certain procedures in which infectious aerosols are created are conducted in biological safety cabinets or other physical containment equipment.

The following standard and special practices, safety equipment and facilities apply to agents assigned to BSL2:

A. *Standard Microbiological Practices*

1. Access to the laboratory is limited or restricted by the laboratory director when work with infectious agents is in progress.
2. Work surfaces are decontaminated at least once a day and after any spill of viable material.
3. All infectious liquid or solid wastes are decontaminated before disposal.
4. Mechanical pipetting devices are used; mouth pipetting is prohibited.
5. Eating, drinking, smoking, and applying cosmetics are not permitted in the work area. Food may be stored in cabinets or refrigerators designated and used for this purpose only. Food storage cabinets or refrigerators should be located outside the work area.
6. Persons must wash their hands after handling infectious materials and animals, and when they leave the laboratory.
7. All procedures are performed carefully to minimize the creation of aerosols.

B. *Special Practices*

1. Contaminated materials that are to be decontaminated at a site away from the laboratory are placed in a durable leak-proof container which is closed before being removed from the laboratory.
2. The laboratory director limits access to the laboratory. In general, persons who are at increased risk of acquiring infection, or for whom infection may be unusually hazardous, are not allowed in the laboratory or animal rooms. The director has the final responsibility for assessing each cir-

cumstance and determining who may enter or work in the laboratory.

3. The laboratory director establishes policies and procedures whereby only persons who have been advised of the potential hazard and who meet any specific entry requirements (e.g., immunization) may enter the laboratory or animal rooms.

4. When the infectious agent(s) in use in the laboratory require special provisions for entry (e.g., vaccination), a hazard warning sign — incorporating the universal biohazard symbol — is posted on the access door to the laboratory work area. The hazard warning sign identifies the infectious agent, lists the name and telephone number of the laboratory director or other responsible person(s), and indicates the special requirement(s) for entering the laboratory.

5. An insect and rodent control program is in effect.

6. Laboratory coats, gowns, smocks, or uniforms are worn while in the laboratory. Before leaving the laboratory for a non-laboratory area (e.g., cafeteria, library, administrative offices), this protective clothing is removed and left in the laboratory or covered with a clean coat not used in the laboratory.

7. Animals not involved in the work being performed are not permitted in the laboratory.

8. Special care is taken to avoid skin contamination with infectious materials; gloves should be worn when handling infected animals and when skin contact with infectious materials is unavoidable.

9. All wastes from laboratories and animal rooms are appropriately decontaminated before disposal.

10. Hypodermic needles and syringes are used only for parenteral injection and aspiration of fluids from laboratory animals and diaphragm bottles. Only needle-locking syringes or disposable syringe-needle units (i.e., needle is integral to the syringe) are used for the injection or aspiration of infectious fluids. Extreme caution should be used when handling needles and syringes to avoid autoinoculation and the generation of aerosols during use and disposal. Needles should not be bent, sheared, replaced in the sheath or guard or removed from the syringe following use. The needle and syringe should be placed promptly in a puncture-resistant container and decontaminated, preferably by autoclaving, before discard or reuse.

11. Spills and accidents that result in overt exposures to infectious materials are immediately reported to the laboratory director. Medical evaluation, surveillance, and treatment are provided as appropriate and written records are maintained.

12. When appropriate, considering the agent(s) handled, baseline serum samples for laboratory and other at-risk personnel are collected and stored. Additional serum specimens may be collected periodically, depending on the agents handled or the function of the facility.

13. A biosafety manual is prepared or adopted. Personnel are advised of special hazards and are required to read instructions on practices and procedures and to follow them.

C. *Containment Equipment*

Biological safety cabinets (Class I or II) or other appropriate personal protective or physical containment devices are used whenever:

1. Procedures with a high potential for creating infectious aerosols are conducted. These may include centrifuging, grinding, blending, vigorous shaking or mixing, sonic disruption, opening containers of infectious materials whose internal pressures may be different from ambient pressures, inoculating animals intranasally, and harvesting infected tissues from animals or eggs.

2. High concentrations or large volumes of infectious agents are used. Such materials may be centrifuged in the open laboratory if sealed heads or centrifuge safety cups are used and if they are opened only in a biological safety cabinet.

D. *Laboratory Facilities*

1. The laboratory is designed so it can be cleaned easily.

2. Bench tops are impervious to water and resistant to acids, alkalis, organic solvents, and moderate heat.

3. Laboratory furniture is study, and spaces between benches, cabinets and equipment are accessible for cleaning.

4. Each laboratory contains a sink for handwashing.

5. If the laboratory has windows that open, they are fitted with fly screens.
6. An autoclave for decontaminating infectious laboratory wastes is available.

Biosafety Level 3 (BSL3) is applicable to clinical, diagnostic, teaching, research, or production facilities in which work is done with indigenous or exotic agents that may cause serious or potentially lethal disease as a result of exposure by the inhalation route. Laboratory personnel have specific training in handling pathogenic and potentially lethal agents and are supervised by competent scientists who are experienced in working with these agents. All procedures involving the manipulation of infectious material are conducted within biological safety cabinets or other physical containment devices, or by personnel wearing appropriate personal protective clothing and devices. The laboratory has special engineering and design features. It is recognized, however, that many existing facilities might not have all the facility safeguards recommended for BSL3 (e.g., access zone, sealed penetrations, and directional airflow, etc.). In these circumstances, acceptable safety may be achieved for routine or repetitive operations (e.g., diagnostic procedures involving the propagation of an agent for identification, typing, and susceptibility testing) in laboratories where facility features satisfy BSL2 recommendations, provided the recommended "Standard Microbiological Practices," "Special Practices," and "Containment Equipment" for BSL3 are rigorously followed. The decision to implement this modification of BSL3 recommendations should be made only by the laboratory director.

The following standard and special safety practices, equipment and facilities apply to agents assigned to BSL3:

A. *Standard Microbiological Practices*

1. Work surfaces are decontaminated at least once a day and after any spill of viable material.
2. All infectious liquid or solid wastes are decontaminated before disposal.
3. Mechanical pipetting devices are used; mouth pipetting is prohibited.
4. Eating, drinking, smoking, storing food, and applying cosmetics are not permitted in the work area.
5. Persons wash their hands after handling infectious materials and animals, and when they leave the laboratory.
6. All procedures are performed carefully to minimize the creation of aerosols.

B. *Special Practices*

1. Laboratory doors are kept closed when experiments are in progress.
2. Contaminated materials that are to be decontaminated at a site away from the laboratory are placed in a durable, leak-proof container which is closed before being removed from the laboratory.
3. The laboratory director limits access to the laboratory and restricts access to persons whose presence is required for program or support purposes. Persons who are at increased risk of acquiring infection, or for whom infection might be unusually hazardous, are not allowed in the laboratory or animal rooms. The director has the final responsibility for assessing each circumstance and determining who may enter or work in the laboratory.
4. The laboratory director establishes policies and procedures whereby only persons who have been advised of the potential biohazard, who meet any specific entry requirements (e.g., immunization), and who comply with all entry and exit procedures may enter the laboratory or animal rooms.
5. When infectious materials or infected animals are present in the laboratory or containment module, a hazard warning sign — incorporating the universal biohazard symbol — is posted on all laboratory and animal room access doors. The hazard warning sign identifies the infectious agent, lists the name and telephone number of the laboratory director or other responsible person(s), and indicates any special requirement(s) for entering the laboratory, such as the need for immunizations, respirators, or other personal protective measures.
6. All activities involving infectious materials are conducted in biological safety cabinets or other physical containment devices within the containment module. No work in open vessels is conducted on the open bench.

7. The work surfaces of biological safety cabinets and other containment equipment are decontaminated when work with infectious materials is finished. Plastic-backed paper toweling used on nonperforated work surfaces within biological safety cabinets facilitates cleanup.
8. An insect and rodent control program is in effect.
9. Laboratory clothing that protects street clothing (e.g., solid front or wrap-around gowns, scrub suits, coveralls) is worn in the laboratory. Laboratory clothing is not worn outside the laboratory, and it is decontaminated before being laundered.
10. Special care is taken to avoid skin contamination with infectious materials; gloves should be worn when handling infected animals and when skin contact with infectious materials is unavoidable.
11. Molded surgical masks or respirators are worn in rooms containing infected animals.
12. Animals not involved in the work being conducted are not permitted in the laboratory.
13. All wastes from laboratories and animal rooms are appropriately decontaminated before disposal.
14. Vacuum lines are protected with high-efficiency particulate air (HEPA) filters and liquid disinfectant traps.
15. Hypodermic needles and syringes are used only for parenteral injection and aspiration of fluids from laboratory animals and diaphragm bottles. Only needle-locking syringes or disposable syringe-needle units (i.e., needle is integral to the syringe) are used for the injection or aspiration of infectious fluids. Extreme caution should be used when handling needles and syringes to avoid autoinoculation and the generation of aerosols during use and disposal. Needles should not be bent, sheared, replaced in the sheath or guard or removed from the syringe following use. The needle and syringe should be placed promptly in a puncture-resistant container and decontaminated, preferably by autoclaving, before discard or reuse.
16. Spills and accidents that result in overt exposures to infectious materials are reported immediately to the laboratory director. Appropriate medical evaluation, surveillance and treatment are provided and written records are maintained.
17. Baseline serum samples for all laboratory and other at-risk personnel should be collected and stored. Additional serum specimens may be collected periodically, depending on the agents handled or the function of the laboratory.
18. A biosafety manual is prepared or adopted. Personnel are advised of special hazards and are required to read instructions on practices and procedures and to follow them.

C. *Containment Equipment*

Biological safety cabinets (Class I or II) or other appropriate combinations of personal protective or physical containment devices (e.g., special protective clothing, masks, gloves, respirators, centrifuge safety cups, sealed centrifuge rotors, and containment caging for animals) are used for all activities with infectious materials that pose a threat of aerosol exposure. These include manipulation of cultures and of those clinical or environmental materials that might be a source of infectious aerosols, the aerosol challenge of experimental animals; harvesting of tissues or fluids from infected animals and embryonated eggs; and necropsy of infected animals.

D. *Laboratory Facilities*

1. The laboratory is separated from areas that are open to unrestricted traffic flow within the building. Passage through two sets of doors is the basic requirement for entry into the laboratory from access corridors or other contiguous areas. Physical separation of the high containment laboratory from access corridors or other laboratories or activities may also be provided by a double-doored clothes change room (showers may be included), airlock, or other access facility that requires passage through two sets of doors before entering the laboratory.
2. The interior surfaces of walls, floors, and ceilings are water-resistant so they can be cleaned easily. Penetrations in these surfaces are sealed or capable of being sealed to facilitate decontaminating the area.
3. Bench tops are impervious to water and resistant to acids, alkalis, organic solvents, and moderate heat.

4. Laboratory furniture is sturdy, and spaces between benches, cabinets, and equipment are accessible for cleaning.
5. Each laboratory contains a sink for handwashing. The sink is foot, elbow, or automatically operated and is located near the laboratory exit door.
6. Windows in the laboratory are closed and sealed.
7. Access doors to the laboratory or containment module are self-closing.
8. An autoclave for decontaminating infectious laboratory wastes is available.
9. A ducted exhaust air ventilation system is provided. This system creates directional airflow that draws air into the laboratory through the entry areas. The exhaust air is not re-circulated to any other area of the building, is discharged to the outside, and is dispersed away from occupied areas and air intakes. Personnel must verify that the direction of the airflow (into the laboratory) is proper. The exhaust air from the laboratory room can be discharged to the outside without being filtered or otherwise treated.
10. The HEPA-filtered exhaust air from Class I or Class II biological safety cabinets is discharged directly to the outside or through the building exhaust system. Exhaust air from Class I or II biological safety cabinets may be re-circulated within the laboratory if the cabinet is tested and certified at least every 12 months. If the HEPA-filtered exhaust air from Class I or II biological safety cabinets is to be discharged to the outside through the building exhaust air system, it is connected to this system in a manner (e.g., thimble unit connection) that avoids any interference with the air balance of the cabinets or building exhaust system.

Biosafety Level 4 (BSL4) is required for work with dangerous and exotic agents that pose a high individual risk of life-threatening disease. Members of the laboratory staff have specific and thorough training in handling extremely hazardous infectious agents, and they understand the primary and secondary containment functions of the standard and special practices, the containment equipment, and the laboratory design characteristics. They are supervised by competent scientists who are trained and experienced in working with these agents. Access to the laboratory is strictly controlled by the laboratory director. The facility is either in a separate building or in a controlled area within a building, which is completely isolated from all other areas of the building. A specific facility operations manual is prepared or adopted.

Within work areas of the facility, all activities are confined to Class III biological safety cabinets or Class I or Class II biological safety cabinets used along with one-piece, positive-pressure, personnel suits ventilated by a life support system. The maximum containment laboratory has special engineering and design features to prevent microorganisms from being disseminated into the environment.

The following standard and special safety practices, equipment, and facilities apply to agents assigned to BSL4:

A. *Standard Microbiological Practices*

1. Work surfaces are decontaminated at least once a day and immediately after any spill of viable material.
2. Only mechanical pipetting devices are used.
3. Eating, drinking, smoking, storing food, and applying cosmetics are not permitted in the laboratory.
4. All procedures are performed carefully to minimize the creation of aerosols.

B. *Special Practices*

1. Biological materials to be removed from the Class III cabinet or from the maximum containment laboratory in a viable or intact state are transferred to a nonbreakable, sealed primary container and then enclosed in a nonbreakable, sealed secondary container which is removed from the facility through a disinfectant dunk tank, fumigation chamber, or an airlock designed for this purpose.
2. No materials, except for biological materials that are to remain in a viable or intact state, are removed from the maximum containment laboratory unless they have been autoclaved or decontaminated before they leave the facility. Equipment or material that might be damaged by high temperatures or steam is decontaminated by gaseous or vapor methods in an airlock or chamber designed for this purpose.

3. Only persons whose presence in the facility or individual laboratory rooms is required for program or support purposes are authorized to enter. Persons who may be at increased risk of acquiring infection, or for whom infection may be unusually hazardous, are not allowed in the laboratory or animal rooms. The supervisor has the final responsibility for assessing each circumstance and determining who may enter or work in the laboratory. Access to the facility is limited by means of secure, locked doors; accessibility is managed by the laboratory director, biohazards control officer, or other person responsible for the physical security of the facility. Before entering, persons are advised of the potential biohazards and instructed as to appropriate safeguards for ensuring their safety. Authorized persons comply with the instructions and all other applicable entry and exit procedures. A logbook signed by all personnel, indicates the date and time of each entry and exit. Practical and effective protocols for emergency situations are established.
4. Personnel enter and leave the facility only through the clothing change and shower rooms. Personnel shower each time they leave the facility. Personnel use the airlocks to enter or leave the laboratory only in an emergency.
5. Street clothing is removed in the outer clothing change room and kept there. Complete laboratory clothing (including undergarments, pants and shirts or jumpsuits, shoes, and gloves) is provided and used by all personnel entering the facility. Head covers are provided for personnel who do not wash their hair during the exit shower. When leaving the laboratory and before proceeding into the shower area, personnel remove their laboratory clothing and store it in a locker or hamper in the inner change room.
6. When infectious materials or infected animals are present in the laboratory or animal rooms, a hazard warning sign — incorporating the universal biohazard symbol — is posted on all access doors. The sign identifies the agent, lists the name of the laboratory director or other responsible person(s), and indicates any special requirements for entering the area (e.g., the need for immunizations or respirators).
7. Supplies and materials needed in the facility are brought in by way of the double-doored autoclave, fumigation chamber, or airlock which is appropriately decontaminated between each use. After securing the outer doors, personnel within the facility retrieve the materials by opening the interior doors of the autoclave, fumigation chamber, or airlock. These doors are secured after materials are brought into the facility.
8. An insect and rodent control program is in effect.
9. Materials (e.g., plants, animals, and clothing) not related to the experiment being conducted are not permitted in the facility.
10. Hypodermic needles and syringes are used only for parenteral injection and aspiration of fluids from laboratory animals and diaphragm bottles. Only needle-locking syringes or disposable syringe-needle units (i.e., needle is integral to the syringe) are used for the injection or aspiration of infectious fluids. Needles should not be bent, sheared, replaced in the sheath or guard or removed from the syringe following use. The needle and syringe should be placed promptly in a puncture-resistant container and decontaminated, preferably by autoclaving, before discard or reuse. Whenever possible, cannulas are used instead of sharp needles (e.g., gavage).
11. A system is set up for reporting laboratory accidents and exposures and employee absenteeism, and for the medical surveillance of potential laboratory-associated illnesses. Written records are prepared and maintained. An essential adjunct to such a reporting-surveillance system is the availability of a facility for the quarantine, isolation, and medical care of personnel with potential or known laboratory-associated illnesses.

C. *Containment Equipment*

All procedures within the facility with agents assigned to BSL4 are conducted in the Class III biological safety cabinet or in Class I or II biological safety cabinets used in conjunction with one-piece, positive-pressure personnel suits ventilated by a life support system. Activities with viral agents (e.g., Rift Valley fever virus) that require BSL4 secondary containment capabilities, and for which highly effective vaccines are available and used, can be conducted within Class I or Class II biological safety cabinets within the facility without the one-piece, positive-pressure personnel suit being used if 1) the facility has been decontaminated; 2) no work is being conducted in the facility with other agents assigned to BSL4; and 3) all other standard and special practices are followed.

D. *Laboratory Facilities*

1. The maximum containment facility consists of either a separate building or a clearly demarcated and isolated zone within a building. Outer and inner change rooms separated by a shower are provided for personnel entering and leaving the facility. A double-doored autoclave, fumigation chamber or ventilated airlock is provided for passage of those materials, supplies, or equipment that are not brought into the facility through the change room.

2. Walls, floors, and ceilings of the facility are constructed to form a sealed internal shell which facilitates fumigation and is animal- and insect-proof. The internal surfaces of this shell are resistant to liquids and chemicals, thus facilitating cleaning and decontamination of the area. All penetrations in these structures and surfaces are sealed. Any drains in the floors contain traps filled with a chemical disinfectant of demonstrated efficacy against the target agent, and they are connected directly to the liquid waste decontamination system. Sewer and other ventilation lines contain HEPA filters.

3. Internal facility appurtenances (such as light fixtures, air ducts, and utility pipes) are arranged to minimize the horizontal surface area on which dust can settle.

4. Bench tops have seamless surfaces that are impervious to water and resistant to acids, alkalis, organic solvents, and moderate heat.

5. Laboratory furniture is of simple and sturdy construction, and spaces between benches, cabinets, and equipment are accessible for cleaning.

6. A foot-, elbow-, or automatically operated handwashing sink is provided near the door of each laboratory room in the facility.

7. If there is a central vacuum system, it does not serve areas outside the facility. In-line HEPA filters are placed as near as practicable to each use point or service cock. Filters are installed to permit in-place decontamination and replacement. Other liquid and gas services to the facility are protected by devices that prevent backflow.

8. If water fountains are provided, they are foot-operated and are located in the facility corridors outside the laboratory. The water service to the fountain is not connected to the backflow-protected distribution system supplying water to the laboratory areas.

9. Access doors to the laboratory are self-closing and lockable.

10. Any windows are breakage-resistant.

11. A double-doored autoclave is provided for decontaminating materials passing out of the facility. The autoclave door that opens to the area external to the facility is sealed to the outer wall and automatically controlled so that the outside door can be opened only after the autoclave "sterilization" cycle has been completed.

12. A pass-through dunk tank, fumigation chamber, or an equivalent decontamination method is provided so that materials and equipment that cannot be decontaminated in the autoclave can be safely removed from the facility.

13. Liquid effluents from laboratory sinks, biological safety cabinets, floors, and autoclave chambers are decontaminated by heat treatment before being released from the maximum containment facility. Liquid wastes from shower rooms and toilets may be decontaminated with chemical disinfectants or by heat in the liquid waste decontamination system. The procedure used for heat decontamination of liquid wastes is evaluated mechanically and biologically by using a recording thermometer and an indicator microorganism with a defined heat susceptibility pattern. If liquid wastes from the shower rooms are decontaminated with chemical disinfectants, the chemical used is of demonstrated efficacy against the target or indicator microorganisms.

14. An individual supply and exhaust air ventilation system is provided. The system maintains pressure differentials and directional airflow as required to assure flow inward from areas outside of the facility toward areas of highest potential risk within the facility. Manometers are used to sense pressure differentials between adjacent areas maintained at different pressure levels. If a system malfunctions, the manometers sound an alarm. The supply and exhaust airflow is interlocked to assure inward (or zero) airflow at all times.

15. The exhaust air from the facility is filtered through HEPA filters and discharged to the outside so that it is dispersed away from occupied buildings and air intakes. Within the facility, the filters are located as near the laboratories as practicable to reduce the length of potentially contaminated air ducts. The filter chambers are designed to allow *in situ* decontamination before filters are removed, and to facilitate certification testing after they are replaced. Coarse filters and HEPA filters are provided to treat air supplied to the facility to increase the lifetime of the exhaust HEPA filters and to protect the supply air system in case air pressures become unbalanced in the laboratory.

16. The treated exhaust air from Class I and II biological safety cabinets can be discharged into the laboratory room environment or to the outside through the facility air exhaust system. If exhaust air from Class I or II biological safety cabinets is discharged into the laboratory, the cabinets are tested and certified at six-month intervals. The treated exhausted air from Class III biological safety cabinets is discharged, without recirculation, through two sets of HEPA filters in series, via the facility exhaust air system. If the treated exhaust air from any of these cabinets is discharged to the outside through the facility exhaust air system, it is connected to this system in a manner (e.g., thimble unit connection) that avoids any interference with the air balance of the cabinets or the facility exhaust air system.

17. A specially designed suit area may be provided in the facility. Personnel who enter this area wear a one-piece, positive-pressure suit that is ventilated by a life support system. The life support system includes alarms and emergency backup breathing air tanks. Entry to this area is through an airlock fitted with airtight doors. A chemical shower is provided to decontaminate the surface of the suit before the worker leaves the area. The exhaust air from the suit area is filtered by two sets of HEPA filters installed in series. A duplicate filtration unit, exhaust fan, and an automatically starting emergency power source are provided. The air pressure within the suit area is lower than that of any adjacent area. Emergency lighting and communication systems are provided. All penetrations into the internal shell of the suit area are sealed. A double-doored autoclave is provided for decontaminating waste materials to be removed from the suit area.

Appendix III

Biosafety Level Criteria for Vertebrate Animals *

If experimental animals are used, institutional management must provide facilities and staff and establish practices that reasonably ensure appropriate levels of environmental quality, safety, and care. Laboratory animal facilities are extensions of the laboratory and, in some situations, are integral to and inseparable from the laboratory. As a general principle, the biosafety level (facilities, practices, and operational requirements) recommended for working with infectious agents *in vivo* and *in vitro* are comparable. The essential elements of the four biosafety levels for activities involving vertebrate animals are summarized in Table I below.

These recommendations presuppose that laboratory animal facilities, operational practices, and quality of animal care meet applicable standards and regulations, and that appropriate species have been selected for animal experiments (e.g., according to NIH's *Guide for the Care and Use of Laboratory Animals*[1] and "Laboratory Animal Welfare Regulations," 9 CFR, Subchapter A, Parts 1, 2, and 3.)

Ideally, facilities for laboratory animals used for studies of infectious or noninfectious disease should be physically separate from other activities such as animal production and quarantine; clinical laboratories; and especially from facilities that provide patient care. Animal facilities should be designed and constructed to facilitate cleaning and housekeeping. A "clean hall/dirty hall" layout is very useful in reducing cross-contamination. Floor drains should be installed in animal facilities only on the basis of clearly defined needs. If floor drains are installed, the drain traps should always contain water.

Table I. Summary of Recommended Biosafety Levels for Activities in which Experimentally or Naturally Infected Vertebrate Animals are Used

Biosafety Level	Practices and Techniques	Safety Equipment	Facilities
1	Standard animal care and management practices	None	Basic
2	Laboratory coats; decontamination of all infectious wastes; limited access; protective gloves and biohazard warning signs as indicated.	Partial containment equipment and/or personal protective devices used for activities and manipulations of agents or infected animals that produce aerosols.	Basic
3	Level 2 practices, plus: special laboratory clothing; controlled access.	Partial containment equipment used for all manipulations of infectious material.	Containment
4	Level 3 practices, plus: entrance through clothes-change room where street clothing is removed and laboratory clothing is put on; shower on exit; all wastes are decontaminated before removal from the facility.	Maximum containment equipment (i.e., Class III biological safety cabinet or partial containment equipment in combination with full-body, air-supplied, positive-pressure personnel suit) used for all procedures and activities.	Maximum Containment

---

* Adapted from *Biosafety in Microbiological and Biomedical Laboratories*, 3rd Ed., USDHHS, USPHS, CDC, NIH, May 1993.

These recommendations describe four combinations of practices, safety equipment, and facilities for experiments on animals infected with agents known or believed to produce infections in humans. These four combinations provide increasing levels of protection to personnel and to the environment, and are recommended as minimal standards for activities involving infected laboratory animals. These four combinations, designated animal biosafety levels (ABSL) 1–4, describe animal facilities and practices applicable to work on animals infected with agents assigned to corresponding biosafety levels (BSL) 1–4.

Facility standards and practices for invertebrate vectors and hosts are not addressed specifically in standards written for commonly used laboratory animals. "Laboratory Safety for Arboviruses and Certain Other Viruses of Vertebrates" — prepared by the Subcommittee on Arbovirus Laboratory Safety of the American Committee on Arthropod-Borne Viruses — serves as a useful reference in the design and operation of facilities using arthropods.[2]

Animal Biosafety Level 1:

A. *Standard Practices*

1. Doors to animal rooms open inward, are self-closing, and are kept closed when experimental animals are present.
2. Work surfaces are decontaminated after use or after any spill of viable materials.
3. Eating, drinking, smoking, and storing food for human use are not permitted in animal rooms.
4. Personnel wash their hands after handling cultures and animals and before leaving the animal room.
5. All procedures are performed carefully to minimize the creation of aerosols.
6. An insect and rodent control program is in effect.

B. *Special Practices*

1. Bedding materials from animal cages are removed in such a manner to minimize the creation of aerosols and are disposed of in compliance with applicable institutional or local requirements.
2. Cages are washed manually or in a cagewasher. Temperature of final rinse water in a mechanical washer should be 180°F.
3. The wearing of laboratory coats, gowns, or uniforms in the animal room is recommended. It is further recommended that laboratory coats worn in the animal room not be worn in other areas.

C. *Containment Equipment*

Special containment equipment is not required for animals infected with agents assigned to BSL1.

D. *Animal Facilities*

1. The animal facility is designed and constructed to facilitate cleaning and housekeeping.
2. A handwashing sink is available in the animal facility.
3. If the animal facility has windows that open, they are fitted with fly screens.
4. It is recommended, but not required, that the direction of airflow in the animal facility is inward and that exhaust air is discharged to the outside without being recirculated to other rooms.

Animal Biosafety Level 2:

A. *Standard Practices*

1. Doors to animal rooms open inward, are self-closing, and are kept closed when infected animals are present.
2. Work surfaces are decontaminated after use or spills of viable materials.
3. Eating, drinking, smoking, and storing of food for human use are not permitted in animal rooms.
4. Personnel wash their hands after handing cultures and animals, and before leaving the animal room.
5. All procedures are performed carefully to minimize the creation of aerosols.
6. An insect and rodent control program is in effect.

B. *Special Practices*

1. Cages are decontaminated, preferably by autoclaving, before they are cleaned and washed.
2. Surgical-type masks are worn by all personnel entering animal rooms housing nonhuman primates.
3. Laboratory coats, gowns, or uniforms are worn while in the animal room. This protective clothing is removed before leaving the animal facility.
4. The laboratory or animal facility director limits access to the animal room to personnel who have been advised of the potential hazard and who need to enter the room for program or service purposes when work is in progress. In general, persons who may be at increased risk of acquiring infection or for whom infection might be unusually hazardous are not allowed in the animal room.
5. The laboratory or animal facility director establishes policies and procedures whereby only persons who have been advised of the potential hazard and meet any specific requirements (e.g., for immunization) may enter the animal room.
6. When the infectious agent(s) in use in the animal room requires special entry provisions (e.g., vaccination), a hazard warning sign — incorporating the universal biohazard symbol — is posted on the access door to the animal room. The hazard warning sign identifies the infectious agent, lists the name and telephone number of the animal facility supervisor or other responsible person(s), and indicates the special requirement(s) for entering the animal room.
7. Special care is taken to avoid skin contamination with infectious materials; gloves should be worn when handling infected animals and when skin contact with infectious materials is unavoidable.
8. All wastes from the animal room are appropriately decontaminated — preferably by autoclaving — before disposal. Infected animal carcasses are incinerated after being transported from the animal room in leakproof, covered containers.
9. Hypodermic needles and syringes are used only for the parenteral injection or aspiration of fluids from laboratory animals and diaphragm bottles. Only needle-locking syringes or disposable needle syringe units (i.e., the needle is integral to the syringe) are used for the injection or aspiration of infectious fluids. Needles should not be bent, sheared, replaced in the sheath or guard, or removed from the syringe following use. The needle and syringe should be placed promptly in a puncture-resistant container and decontaminated — preferably by autoclaving — before being discarded or reused.
10. If floor drains are provided, the drain traps shall always be filled with water or a suitable disinfectant.
11. When appropriate, considering the agents handled, baseline serum samples from animal care and other at-risk personnel are collected and stored. Additional serum samples may be collected periodically, depending on the agents handled or the function of the facility.

C. *Containment Equipment*

Biological safety cabinets, other physical containment devices, and/or personal protective devices (e.g., respirators, face shields) are used whenever procedures with a high potential for creating aerosols are conducted. These include necropsy of infected animals; harvesting of infected tissues or fluids from animals or eggs; intranasal inoculation of animals; and manipulations of high concentrations or large volumes of infectious materials.

D. *Animal Facilities*

1. The animal facility is designed and constructed to facilitate cleaning and housekeeping.
2. A handwashing sink is available in the room where infected animals are housed.
3. If the animal facility has windows that open, they are fitted with fly screens.
4. It is recommended, but not required, that the direction of airflow in the animal facility is inward and that exhaust air is discharged to the outside without being recirculated to other rooms.
5. An autoclave that can be used for decontaminating infectious laboratory waste is available in the building with the animal facility.

Animal Biosafety Level 3:

A. *Standard Practices*

1. Doors to animal rooms open inward, are self-closing, and are kept closed when work with infected animals is in progress.

2. Work surfaces are decontaminated after use or spills of viable materials.
3. Eating, drinking, smoking, and storing of food for human use are not permitted in animal rooms.
4. Personnel wash their hands after handing cultures and animals, and before leaving the animal room.
5. All procedures are performed carefully to minimize the creation of aerosols.
6. An insect and rodent control program is in effect.

B. *Special Practices*

1. Cages are autoclaved before bedding is removed and before they are cleaned and washed.
2. Surgical-type masks or other respiratory protection devices (e.g., respirators) are worn by personnel entering animal rooms housing animals infected with agents assigned to BSL3.
3. Wrap-around or solid-front gowns or uniforms are worn by personnel entering the animal room. Front-button laboratory coats are unsuitable. Protective gowns must remain in the animal room and must be decontaminated before being laundered.
4. The laboratory director or other responsible person restricts access to the animal room to personnel who have been advised of the potential hazard and who need to enter the room for program or service purposes when infected animals are present. In general, persons who may be at increased risk of acquiring infection, or for whom infection might be unusually hazardous, are not allowed in the animal room.
5. The laboratory director or other responsible person establishes policies and procedures whereby only persons who have been advised of the potential hazard and meet any specific requirements (e.g., for immunization) may enter the animal room.
6. Hazard warning signs — incorporating the universal biohazard warning symbol — are posted on access doors to animal rooms containing animals infected with agents assigned to BSL3. The hazard warning sign should identify the agent(s) in use, list the name and telephone number of the animal room supervisor or other responsible person(s), and indicate any special conditions of entry into the animal room (e.g., the need for immunizations or respirators).
7. Personnel wear gloves when handling infected animals. Gloves are removed aseptically and autoclaved with other animal room wastes before being disposed of or reused.
8. All wastes from the animal room are autoclaved before disposal. All animal carcasses are incinerated. Dead animals are transported from the animal room to the incinerator in leakproof, covered containers.
9. Hypodermic needles and syringes are used only for gavage or for parenteral injection or aspiration of fluids from laboratory animals and diaphragm bottles. Only needle-locking syringes or disposable needle syringe units (i.e., the needle is integral to the syringe) are used. Needles should not be bent, sheared, replaced in the sheath or guard, or removed from the syringe following use. The needle and syringe should be placed promptly in a puncture-resistant container and decontaminated — preferably by autoclaving — before being discarded or reused. Whenever possible, cannulas should be used instead of sharp needles (e.g., gavage).
10. If floor drains are provided, the drain traps shall always be filled with water or a suitable disinfectant.
11. If vacuum lines are provided, they should be protected with high-efficiency particulate air (HEPA) filters and liquid disinfectant traps.
12. Boots, shoe covers, or other protective footwear and disinfectant footbaths are available and used when indicated.

C. *Containment Equipment*

1. Personal protective clothing and equipment and/or other physical containment devices are used for all procedures and manipulations of infectious materials or infected animals.
2. The risk of infectious aerosols from infected animals or their bedding can be reduced if animals are housed in partial containment caging systems, such as open cages placed in ventilated enclosures (e.g., laminar flow cabinets); solid wall and bottom cages covered by filter bonnets; or other equivalent primary containment systems.

D. *Animal Facilities*

1. The animal facility is designed and constructed to facilitate cleaning and housekeeping, and is separated from areas that are open to unrestricted personnel traffic within the building. Passage

through two sets of doors is the basic requirement for entry into the animal room from access corridors or other contiguous areas. Physical separation of the animal room from access corridors or other activities may also be provided by a double-doored clothes change room (showers may be included), airlock, or other access facility that requires passage through two sets of doors before entering the animal room.

2. The interior surfaces of walls, floors, and ceilings are water-resistant so that they may be easily cleaned. Penetrations in these surfaces are sealed, or capable of being sealed, to facilitate fumigation or space decontamination.
3. A foot-, elbow-, or automatically operated handwashing sink is provided near each animal room exit door.
4. Windows in the animal room are closed and sealed.
5. Animal room doors are self-closing and are kept closed when infected animals are present.
6. An autoclave for decontaminating waste is available, preferably within the animal room. Materials to be autoclaved outside the animal room are transported in a leakproof, covered container.
7. An exhaust air ventilation system is provided. This system creates directional airflow that draws air into the animal room through the entry area. The building exhaust can be used for this purpose if the exhaust air is not recirculated to any other area of the building, is discharged to the outside, and is dispersed away from occupied areas and air intakes. Personnel must verify that the direction of the airflow (into the animal room) is proper. The exhaust air from the animal room that does not pass through biological safety cabinets or other primary containment equipment can be discharged to the outside without being filtered or otherwise treated.
8. The HEPA-filtered exhaust air from Class I or Class II biological safety cabinets or other primary containment devices is discharged directly to the outside or through the building exhaust system. Exhaust air from these primary containment devices may be recirculated within the animal room if the cabinet is tested and certified at least every 12 months. If the HEPA-filtered exhaust air from Class I or Class II biological safety cabinets is discharged to the outside through the building exhaust system, it is connected to this system in a manner (e.g., thimble unit connection) that avoids any interference with the air balance of the cabinets or building exhaust system.

Animal Biosafety Level 4:

A. *Standard Practices*

1. Doors to animal rooms open inward and are self-closing.
2. Work surfaces are decontaminated after use or spills of viable materials.
3. Eating, drinking, smoking, and storing of food for human use are not permitted in animal rooms.
4. All procedures are performed carefully to minimize the creation of aerosols.
5. An insect and rodent control program is in effect.
6. Cages are autoclaved before bedding is removed and before they are cleaned and washed.

B. *Special Practices*

1. Only persons whose entry into the facility or individual animal rooms is required for program or support purposes are authorized to enter. Persons who may be at increased risk of acquiring infection or for whom infection might be unusually hazardous are not allowed in the animal facility. Persons at increased risk may include children, pregnant women, and persons who are immunodeficient or immunosuppressed. The supervisor has the final responsibility for assessing each circumstance and determining who may enter or work in the laboratory. Access to the facility is limited by secure, locked doors; accessibility is controlled by the animal facility supervisor biohazards control officer, or other person responsible for the physical security of the facility. Before entering, persons are advised of the potential biohazards and instructed on appropriate safeguards. Personnel comply with the instructions and all other applicable entry and exit procedures. Practical and effective protocols for emergency situations are established.
2. Personnel enter and leave the facility only through the clothes change and shower rooms. Personnel shower each time they leave the facility. Head covers are provided to personnel who do not wash their hair during the exit shower. Except in an emergency, personnel do not enter or leave the facility through the airlocks.

3. Street clothing is removed in the outer clothing change room and kept there. Complete laboratory clothing (including undergarments, pants and shirts or jumpsuits, shoes, and gloves) are provided and used by all personnel entering the facility. When exiting, personnel remove laboratory clothing and store it in a locker or hamper in the inner change room before entering the shower area.

4. When infectious materials or infected animals are present in the animal rooms, a hazard warning sign — incorporating the universal biohazard symbol — is posted on all access doors. The sign identifies the agent, lists the name and telephone number of the animal facility supervisor or other responsible person(s), and indicates any special conditions of entry into the area (e.g., the need for immunizations and respirators).

5. Supplies and materials to be taken into the facility enter by way of a double-doored autoclave, fumigation chamber, or airlock that is appropriately decontaminated between each use. After securing the outer doors, personnel inside the facility retrieve the materials by opening the interior doors of the autoclave, fumigation chamber, or airlock. This inner door is secured after materials are brought into the facility.

6. Materials (e.g., plants, animals, clothing) not related to the experiment are not permitted in the facility.

7. Hypodermic needles and syringes are used only for gavage or for parenteral injection and aspiration of fluids from laboratory animals and diaphragm bottles. Only needle-locking syringes or disposable needle syringe units (i.e., the needle is integral to the syringe) are used. Needles should not be bent, sheared, replaced in the sheath or guard, or removed from the syringe following use. The needle and syringe should be placed promptly in a puncture-resistant container and decontaminated — preferably by autoclaving — before being discarded or reused. Whenever possible, cannulas should be used instead of sharp needles (e.g., gavage).

8. A system is developed and is operational for the reporting of animal facility accidents and exposures, employee absenteeism, and for the medical surveillance of potential laboratory-associated illnesses. An essential adjunct to such a reporting/surveillance system is the availability of a facility for the quarantine, isolation, and medical care of persons with potential or known laboratory-associated illnesses.

9. Baseline serum samples are collected and stored for all laboratory and other at-risk personnel. Additional serum specimens may be collected periodically, depending on the agents handled or the function of the laboratory.

C. *Containment Equipment*

Laboratory animals, infected with agents assigned to BSL4, are housed in the Class III biological safety cabinet or in partial containment caging systems (such as open cages placed in ventilated enclosures; solid wall and bottom cages covered with filter bonnets; or other equivalent primary containment systems) in specially designed areas in which all personnel are required to wear one-piece, positive-pressure suits ventilated with life-support systems. Animal work with viral agents that require BSL4 secondary containment, and for which highly effective vaccines are available and used, may be conducted with partial containment cages and without the one-piece, positive-pressure personnel suit if 1) the facility has been decontaminated; 2) if no concurrent experiments requiring BSL4 primary and secondary containment are being done in the facility; and 3) if all other standard and special practices are followed.

D. *Animal Facilities*

1. The animal rooms are located in a separate building or in a clearly demarcated and isolated zone within a building. Outer and inner change rooms, separated by a shower, are provided for personnel entering and leaving the facility. A double-doored autoclave, fumigation chamber, or ventilated airlock is provided for passage of materials, supplies, or equipment which are not brought into the facility through the change room.

2. Walls, floors, and ceilings of the facility are constructed to form a sealed internal shell, which facilitates fumigation and is animal- and insect-proof. The internal surfaces of this shell are resistant to liquids and chemicals, thus facilitating cleaning and decontamination of the area. All penetrations in these structures and surfaces are sealed.

3. Internal facility appurtenances (such as light fixtures, air ducts, and utility pipes) are arranged to minimize the horizontal surface area on which dust can settle.
4. A foot-, elbow-, or automatically operated handwashing sink is provided near the door of each animal room within the facility.
5. If there is a central vacuum system, it does not serve areas outside of the facility. The vacuum system has in-line HEPA filters placed as near as practicable to each use-point or service cock. Filters are installed to permit in-place decontamination and replacement. Other liquid and gas services for the facility are protected by devices that prevent backflow.
6. External animal facility doors are self-closing and self-locking.
7. Any windows must be resistant to breakage and must be sealed.
8. A double-doored autoclave is provided for decontaminating materials that leave the facility. The autoclave door that opens to the area external to the facility is controlled automatically so that it can be opened after the autoclave "sterilization" cycle is completed.
9. A pass-through dunk tank, fumigation chamber, or an equivalent decontamination method is provided so that materials and equipment that cannot be decontaminated in the autoclave can be removed safely from the facility.
10. Liquid effluents from laboratory sinks, cabinets, floors, and autoclave chambers are decontaminated by heat treatment before being discharged. Liquid wastes from shower rooms and toilets may be decontaminated with chemical disinfectants or by heat in the liquid waste decontamination system. The procedure used for heat decontamination of liquid wastes must be evaluated mechanically and biologically by using a recording thermometer and an indicator microorganism with a defined heat susceptibility pattern. If liquid wastes from the shower rooms are decontaminated with chemical disinfectants, the chemicals used must have documented efficacy against the target or indicator microorganisms.
11. An individual supply-and-exhaust air ventilation system is provided. The system maintains pressure differentials, and directional airflow is required to assure inflow from areas outside of the facility toward areas of highest potential risk within the facility. Manometers are provided to sense pressure differentials between adjacent areas that are maintained at different pressure levels. The manometers sound an alarm when a system malfunctions. The supply and exhaust airflow is interlocked to assure inward (or zero) airflow at all times.
13. The exhaust air from the facility is filtered by HEPA filters and discharged to the outside so that it is dispersed away from occupied buildings and air intakes. Within the facility, the filters are located as near to the laboratories as practicable in order to reduce the length of potentially contaminated air ducts. The filter chambers are designed to allow *in situ* decontamination before filters are removed and to facilitate certification testing after they are replaced. Coarse filters are provided for treatment of air supplied to the facility to increase the lifetime of the HEPA filters.
14. The treated exhaust air from Class I or Class II biological safety cabinets can be discharged into the animal room environment or to the outside through the facility air exhaust system. If exhaust air from Class I or II biological safety cabinets is discharged into the animal room, the cabinets are tested and certified at six-month intervals. The treated exhaust air from Class III biological safety cabinets is discharged without recirculation via the facility exhaust air system. If the treated exhaust air from any of these cabinets is discharged to the outside through the facility exhaust air system, it is connected to this system in a manner that avoids any interference with the air balance of the cabinets or the facility exhaust air system.
15. A specially designed suit area may be provided in the facility. Personnel who enter this area wear a one-piece, positive-pressure suit that is ventilated by a life-support system. The life-support system is provided with alarms and emergency backup breathing air tanks. Entry to this area is through an airlock fitted with airtight doors. A chemical shower is provided to decontaminate the surface of the suit before the worker leaves the area. The exhaust air from the area in which the suit is used is filtered by two sets of HEPA filters installed in series. A duplicate filtration unit and exhaust fan are provided. An automatically starting emergency power source is provided. The air pressure within the suit area is lower than that of any adjacent area. Emergency lighting and communication systems are provided. All penetrations into the inner shell of the suit area are sealed. A double-doored autoclave is provided for decontaminating waste materials to be removed from the suit area.

References

1. **U.S. Department of Health and Human Services, National Institutes of Health:** *Guide for the Care and Use of Laboratory Animals* (NIH Publication No. 85-23, Rev. 1985). Bethesda, Md.: National Institutes of Health, 1985.

2. **American Committee on Arthropod-Borne Viruses, Subcommittee on Arbovirus Laboratory Safety**: Laboratory Safety for Arboviruses and Certain Other Viruses of Vertebrates. *Am. J. Trop. Med. Hyg. 29(6):*1359-1381 (1980).

Appendix IV

Biosafety Criteria for Large-Scale Experiments and Manufacturing *

In the National Institutes of Health's *Guidelines for Research Involving Recombinant DNA Molecules* four levels of physical contaminant for large-scale uses of recombinant DNA cultures are established in Appendix K, Section III-B-5.[1] Large-scale is defined as research or production involving viable organisms in cultures greater than 10 L. The four established levels are Good Large-Scale Practice (GLSP); Biosafety Level 1–Large Scale (BSL1–LS); Biosafety Level 2–Large Scale (BSL2–LS); and Biosafety Level 3–Large Scale (BSL3–LS). Containment conditions are set that are appropriate for the hazard presented by the organism to workers or the environment. It is important to note that these biosafety levels considered only the hazard presented by the organisms and not the products produced by the organisms.

Good Large-Scale Practice (GLSP): In 1986, the Organisation for Economic Co-operation and Development (OECD) published the concept of good industrial large-scale practice (GILSP).[2] NIH adopted this concept as GLSP in July of 1991. NIH recommends GLSP "for large-scale research or production involving viable, nonpathogenic, and nontoxicogenic recombinant strains derived from host organisms that have an extended history of safe large-scale use."[1] GLSP is also "recommended for organisms such as those included in Appendix C [of the NIH Guidelines] that have built-in environmental limitations that permit optimum growth in the large-scale setting but limited survival without adverse consequences in the environment." For an organism to be considered GLSP, it must meet the following OECD criteria:[2]

1. The host organism should be nonpathogenic, should not contain adventitious agents, and should have an extended history of safe industrial use, or have built-in environmental limitations that permit optimum growth in the industrial setting or limited survival without adverse consequences in the environment.
2. The rDNA-engineered organism should be nonpathogenic, should be as safe in the industrial setting as the host organism, and should be without adverse consequences in the environment.
3. The vector/insert should be well-characterized and free from known harmful sequences; should be limited in size as much as possible to the DNA required to perform the intended function; should not increase the stability of the construct in the environment unless that is a requirement of the intended function; should be poorly mobilizable; and should not transfer any resistance markers to microorganisms not known to acquire them naturally if such acquisition could compromise the use of a drug to control disease agents in human or veterinary medicine or agriculture.

In Appendix K-II of the guidelines, NIH also delineates operating requirements for GLSP as follows:

1. Institutional codes of practice shall be formulated and implemented to assure adequate control of health and safety matters.
2. Written instructions and training of personnel shall be provided to assure that cultures of viable organisms containing recombinant DNA molecules are handled prudently and that the workplace is kept clean and orderly.

---

* Adapted from *Recombinant DNA Safety Considerations* (OECD, 1986); *Guidelines for Research Involving Recombinant DNA Molecules* (NIH, June 1994); and *Safety Considerations for Biotechnology* (OECD, 1992).

3. In the interest of good personal hygiene, facilities (e.g., handwashing sink, shower, changing room) and protective clothing (e.g., uniforms, laboratory coats) shall be provided that are appropriate for the risk of exposure to viable organisms containing recombinant DNA molecules. Also, eating, drinking, smoking, applying cosmetics, and mouth pipetting shall be prohibited in the work area.

4. Cultures of viable organisms containing recombinant DNA molecules shall be handled in facilities intended to safeguard health during work with microorganisms that do not require containment.

5. Discharges containing viable recombinant organisms shall be handled in accordance with applicable governmental environmental regulations.

6. Addition of materials to a system; sample collection; transfer of culture fluids within or between systems; and processing of culture fluids shall be conducted in a manner that maintains employee exposure to viable organisms containing recombinant DNA molecules at a level that does not adversely affect the health and safety of employees.

7. The facility's emergency response plan shall include provisions for handling spills.

In 1992, the OECD published a new document that elaborated on the 1986 GILSP definition.[3] This publication expands the GILSP definition to include other organisms that do not meet the 1986 definition but have been demonstrated to be of low-risk.

Biosafety Level 1–Large Scale (BSL1–LS): NIH recommends the BSL1–LS level of physical containment for rDNA organisms that require BSL1 containment at the laboratory scale but do not qualify for GLSP.

Following are the recommendations for facility design and practice.

1. Spills and accidents that result in overt exposures to organisms containing recombinant DNA molecules are immediately reported to the laboratory director. Medical evaluation, surveillance, and treatment are provided as appropriate, and written records are maintained.

2. Cultures of viable organisms containing recombinant DNA molecules shall be handled in a closed system (e.g., closed vessel used for the propagation and growth of cultures) or other primary containment equipment (e.g., biological safety cabinet containing a centrifuge used to process culture fluids) that is designed to reduce the potential for escape of viable organisms. Volumes less than 10 L may be handled outside of a closed system or other primary containment equipment, provided that all physical containment requirements specified in Appendix G-II-A of the NIH Guidelines are met.

3. Culture fluids (except as allowed in Appendix K-III-D) shall not be removed from a closed system or other primary containment equipment unless the viable organisms containing recombinant DNA molecules have been inactivated by a validated inactivation procedure. A validated inactivation procedure is one that has been demonstrated to be effective using the organism that will serve as the host for propagating the recombinant DNA molecules.

4. Sample collection from a closed system, the addition of materials to a closed system, and the transfer of culture fluids from one closed system to another shall be done in a manner that minimizes the release of aerosols or contamination of exposed surfaces.

5. Exhaust gases removed from a closed system or other primary containment equipment shall be treated by filters that have efficiencies equivalent to high-efficiency particulate air (HEPA) filters or by other equivalent procedures (e.g., incineration) to minimize the release of viable organisms containing recombinant DNA molecules to the environment.

6. A closed system or other primary containment equipment that has contained viable organisms containing recombinant DNA molecules shall not be opened for maintenance or other purposes unless it has been sterilized by a validated sterilization procedure. A validated sterilization procedure is one that has been demonstrated to be effective using the organism that will serve as the host for propagating the recombinant DNA molecules.

7. Emergency plans required by Sections IV-B-2-b-(6) and IV-B-3-c-(3) of the NIH Guidelines shall include methods and procedures for handling large losses of culture on an emergency basis.

Biosafety Level 2–Large Scale (BSL2–LS): NIH recommends the BSL2–LS level of physical containment for rDNA organisms that require BSL2 containment at the laboratory scale.

1. Cultures of viable organisms containing recombinant DNA molecules shall be handled in a closed system (e.g., closed vessel used for the propagation and growth of cultures) or other primary containment equipment (e.g., Class III biological safety cabinet containing a centrifuge used to process culture fluids) that is designed to prevent the escape of viable organisms.

   Volumes less than 10 L may be handled outside of a closed system or other primary containment equipment, provided that all physical containment requirements specified in Appendix G-II-B of the NIH Guidelines are met.

2. Culture fluids (except as allowed in Appendix K-IV-D) shall not be removed from a closed system or other primary containment equipment unless the viable organisms containing recombinant DNA molecules have been inactivated by a validated inactivation procedure. A validated inactivation procedure is one that has been demonstrated to be effective using the organism that will serve as the host for propagating the recombinant DNA molecules.

3. Sample collection from a closed system, the addition of materials to a closed system, and the transfer of cultures fluids from one closed system to another shall be done in a manner that prevents the release of aerosols or contamination of exposed surfaces.

4. Exhaust gases removed from a closed system or other primary containment equipment shall be treated by filters that have efficiencies equivalent to HEPA filters or by other equivalent procedures (e.g., incineration) to prevent the release of viable organisms containing recombinant DNA molecules to the environment.

5. A closed system or other primary containment equipment that has contained viable organisms containing recombinant DNA molecules shall be opened for maintenance or other purposes unless it has been sterilized by a validated sterilization procedure. A validated sterilization procedure is one that has been demonstrated to be effective using the organisms that will serve as the host for propagating the recombinant DNA molecules.

6. Rotating seals and other mechanical devices directly associated with a closed system used for the propagation and growth of viable organisms containing recombinant DNA molecules shall be designed to prevent leakage or shall be fully enclosed in ventilated housings that are exhausted through filters that have efficiencies equivalent to HEPA filters or through other equivalent treatment devices.

7. A closed system used for the propagation and growth of viable organisms containing recombinant DNA molecules and other primary containment equipment used to contain operations involving viable organisms containing sensing devices that monitor the integrity of containment during operations.

8. A closed system used for the propagation and growth of viable organisms containing the recombinant DNA molecules shall be tested for integrity of the containment features using the organism that will serve as the host for propagating recombinant DNA molecules. Testing shall be accomplished prior to the introduction of viable organisms containing recombinant DNA molecules and following modification or replacement of essential containment features. Procedures and methods used in the testing shall be appropriate for the equipment design and for recovery and demonstration of the test organism. Records of tests and results shall be maintained on file.

9. A closed system used for the propagation and growth of viable organisms containing recombinant DNA molecules shall be permanently identified. This identification shall be used in all records reflecting testing, operation, and maintenance and in all documentation relating to use of this equipment for research or production activities involving viable organisms containing recombinant DNA molecules.

10. The universal biohazard symbol (see Chapter 5, Figure 2) shall be posted on each closed system and primary containment equipment when used to contain viable organisms containing recombinant DNA molecules.

11. Emergency plans required by Sections IV-B-2-b-(6) and IV-B-3-c-(3) of the NIH Guidelines shall include methods and procedures for handling large losses of culture on an emergency basis.

Biosafety Level 3–Large Scale (BSL3–LS): NIH recommends the BSL3–LS level of physical containment for rDNA organisms that require BSL3 containment at the laboratory scale.

1. Spills and accidents that result in overt exposures to organisms containing recombinant DNA molecules are immediately reported to the Biological Safety Officer, Institutional Biosafety Committee, NIH/ORDA, and other appropriate authorities (if applicable).

2. Cultures of viable organisms containing recombinant DNA molecules shall be handled in a closed system (e.g., closed vessels used for the propagation and growth of cultures) or other primary containment equipment (e.g., Class III biological safety cabinet containing a centrifuge used to process culture fluids) that is designed to prevent the escape of viable organisms. Volumes less than 10 L may be handled outside of a closed system, provided that all physical containment requirements specified in Appendix G-II-C of the NIH Guidelines are met.

3. Culture fluids (except as allowed in Appendix K-V-D) shall not be removed from a closed system or other primary containment equipment unless the viable organisms containing recombinant DNA molecules have been inactivated by a validated inactivation procedure. A validated inactivation procedure is one that has been demonstrated to be effective using the organisms that will serve as the host for propagating the recombinant DNA molecules.

4. Sample collection from a closed system, the addition of materials to a closed system, and the transfer of culture fluids from one closed system to another shall be done in a manner that prevents the release or aerosols or contamination of exposed surfaces.

5. Exhaust gases removed from a closed system or other primary containment equipment shall be treated by filters that have efficiencies equivalent to HEPA filters or by other equivalent procedures (e.g, incineration) to prevent the release of viable organisms containing recombinant DNA molecules to the environment.

6. A closed system or other primary containment equipment that has contained viable organisms containing recombinant DNA molecules shall not be opened for maintenance or other purposes unless it has been sterilized by a validated sterilization procedure. A validated sterilization procedure is one that has been demonstrated to be effective using the organisms that will serve as the host for propagating the recombinant DNA molecules.

7. A closed system used for the propagation and growth of viable organisms containing recombinant DNA molecules shall be operated so that the space above the culture level will be maintained at a pressure as low as possible, consistent with equipment design, in order to maintain the integrity of containment features.

8. Rotating seals and other mechanical devices associated directly with a closed system used to contain viable organisms containing recombinant DNA molecules shall be designed to prevent leakage or shall be fully enclosed in ventilated housings that are exhausted through filters that have efficiencies equivalent to HEPA filters or through other equivalent treatment devices.

9. A closed system used for the propagation and growth of viable organisms containing recombinant DNA molecules and other primary containment equipment used to contain operations involving viable organisms containing recombinant DNA molecules shall include monitoring or sensing devices that monitor the integrity of containment during operations.

10. A closed system used for the propagation and growth of viable organisms containing recombinant DNA molecules shall be tested for integrity of the containment features using the organisms that will serve as the host for propagating the recombinant DNA molecules. Testing shall be accomplished prior to the introduction of viable organisms containing recombinant DNA molecules and following modification or replacement of essential containment features. Procedures and methods used in the testing shall be appropriate for the equipment design, and for recovery and demonstration of the test organism. Records of tests and results shall be maintained on file.

11. A closed system used for the propagation and growth of viable organisms containing recombinant DNA molecules shall be permanently identified. This identification shall be used in all records reflecting testing, operation, and maintenance and in all documentation relating to the use of this equipment for research production activities involving viable organisms containing recombinant DNA molecules.

12. The universal biohazard symbol shall be posted on each closed system and primary containment equipment when used to contain viable organisms containing recombinant DNA molecules.

13. Emergency plans required by Sections IV-B-2-b-(6) and IV-B-3-c-(3) of the NIH Guidelines shall include methods and procedures for handling large losses of culture on an emergency basis.

14. Closed systems and other primary containment equipment used in handling cultures of viable organisms containing recombinant DNA molecules shall be located within a controlled area that meets the following requirements:

a. The controlled area shall have a separate entry area. The entry area shall be double-doored space such as an air lock, anteroom, or change room that separates the controlled area from the balance of the facility.

b. The surfaces of walls, ceilings, and floors in the controlled area shall be such as to permit ready cleaning and decontamination.

c. Penetrations into the controlled area shall be sealed to permit liquid or vapor phase space decontamination.

d. All utilities and service or process piping and wiring entering the controlled area shall be protected against contamination.

e. Handwashing facilities equipped with foot, elbow, or automatically operated valves shall be located at each major work area and near each primary exit.

f. A shower facility shall be provided. This facility shall be located in close proximity to the controlled area.

g. The controlled area shall be designed to preclude release of culture fluids outside the controlled area in the event of an accident spill or release from the closed system or other primary containment equipment.

h. The controlled area shall have a ventilation system that is capable of controlling air movement. The movement of air shall be from areas of lower contamination potential to areas of higher contamination potential. If the ventilation system provides positive pressure supply air, the system shall operate in a manner that prevents the reversal of the direction of air movement or shall be equipped with an alarm that would be actuated in the event reversal in the direction of air movement were to occur. The exhaust air from the controlled air shall not be recirculated to the areas of the facility. The exhaust air from the controlled air may not be discharged to the outdoors without being HEPA filtered, subjected to thermal oxidation, or otherwise treated to prevent the release of viable organisms.

15. The following personnel and operational practices shall be required:

a. Personnel entry into the controlled area shall be through the entry area specified in Appendix K-V-N-1 of the NIH Guidelines.

b. Persons entering the controlled area shall exchange or cover their personal clothing with work garments such as jumpsuits, laboratory coats, pants and shirts, head covers, and shoes or shoe covers. On exit from the controlled area, the work clothing may be stored in a locker separate from that used for personal clothing or discarded for laundering. Clothing shall be decontaminated before laundering.

c. Entry into the controlled area during periods when work is in progress shall be restricted to those persons required to meet program or support needs. Before entry, all persons shall be informed of the operating practices, emergency procedures, and the nature of the work conducted.

d. Persons under 18 years of age shall not be permitted to enter the controlled area.

e. The universal biohazard symbol shall be posted on entry doors to the controlled area and all internal doors when any work involving the organism is in progress. This includes periods when decontamination procedures are in progress. The sign posted on the entry doors to the controlled area shall include a statement of agents in use and personnel authorized to enter the controlled area.

f. The controlled area shall be kept neat and clean.

g. Eating, drinking, smoking, and storage of food are prohibited in the controlled area.

h. Animals and plants shall be excluded from the controlled area.

i. An effective insect and rodent control program shall be maintained.

j. Access doors to the controlled area shall be kept closed, except as necessary for access, when work is in progress. Serve doors leading directly outdoors shall be sealed and locked when work is in progress.

k. Persons shall wash their hands when leaving the controlled area.

l. Persons working in the controlled area shall be trained in emergency procedures.

m. Equipment and materials required for the management of accidents involving viable organisms containing recombinant DNA molecules shall be available in the controlled area.

n. The controlled area shall be decontaminated in accordance with established procedures following spills or other accidental release of viable organisms containing recombinant DNA molecules.

References

1. **U.S. Department of Health and Human Services, National Institutes of Health:** *Guidelines for Research Involving Recombinant DNA Molecules (NIH Guidelines).* Bethesda, Md.: National Institutes of Health, 1994.

2. **Organisation for Economic Co-operation and Development:** *Recombinant DNA Safety Considerations.* Paris: Organisation for Economic Co-operation and Development, 1986.

3. **Organisation for Economic Co-operation and Development:** *Safety Considerations for Biotechnology.* Paris: Organisation for Economic Co-operation and Development, 1992.

Appendix V

Example of a Generic Bloodborne Pathogens Written Exposure Control Plan

INTRODUCTION

The purpose of this Exposure Control Plan is to establish minimum requirements and procedures for the safety and health of employees who might be occupationally exposed to human blood or other potentially infectious materials. The Occupational Safety and Health Administration (OSHA) has promulgated a specific standard for bloodborne pathogens (29 CFR 1910.1030). The OSHA standard requires an employer to set forth procedures, equipment, personal protective equipment (PPE), and work practices capable of protecting employees from the health hazards presented by skin, eye, mucous membrane, or parenteral contact with blood or potentially infectious materials that might result from an employee's duties.

The following procedures are based on the requirements of the OSHA standard and the most current professional practices of the field of occupational health and safety. A copy of the standard is included in Appendix A of this plan.

STRATEGY

1. This program is designed to reduce the likelihood of illness to employees by implementing specific procedures to be followed when there is potential exposure to human blood and similar infectious materials.
2. The primary objective is to ensure that all individuals at risk are adequately informed about the risks involved, the procedures to follow, and the PPE to use to minimize exposure.
3. Procedures outlined in this plan can be used for all employees who are responsible for performing laboratory procedures.

Definitions

In this plan, all references to "occupational exposure" will mean reasonably anticipated skin, eye, mucous membrane, or parenteral contact with human blood or other potentially infectious materials that might result from an employee's duties. **NOTE:** This definition does *not* cover "Good Samaritan" acts that result in exposure to blood or other potentially infectious materials from assisting a fellow employee, although OSHA encourages employers to offer follow-up procedures in such cases.

"Regulated Waste" means liquid or semi-liquid blood or other potentially infectious materials; contaminated items that would release blood or other potentially infectious materials in a liquid or semi-liquid state if compressed; items that are caked with dried blood or other potentially infectious material and are capable of releasing these materials during handling; contaminated sharps; and pathological or microbiological wastes containing blood or other potentially infectious materials.

For more definitions, consult Paragraph (b) of 29 CFR 1910.1030 (see Appendix A).

RESPONSIBILITIES

- **Management:** It is management's responsibility to develop and implement an exposure control plan. This responsibility includes providing personnel with safe working procedures, handwashing facilities, personal protective equipment, and adequate training on the hazards of human blood and other potentially infectious materials, and the safe work practices to follow when potentially exposed.

  Management must review and evaluate the effectiveness of the site Hazard Control Plan at least annually and update it as necessary.

- **Supervisors:** The supervisors of health and emergency care workers, and supervisors of other workers occupationally exposed, are responsible for the overall application of the plan. Supervisors must ensure that workers know and follow the safe work procedures outlined in the plan, that protective equipment is available, and that appropriate training has been provided.

- **Employees:** It is the responsibility of the occupationally exposed employee to plan and conduct each operation in accordance with the procedures in this plan and to develop good personal work habits. The employee should become familiar with procedures for limiting exposure to human blood and other infectious materials, especially through the use of Universal Precautions — as recommended or defined by the Centers for Disease Control and Prevention (CDC) and/or OSHA — and/or Body Substance Isolation procedures, in addition to the proper use of personal protective equipment.

AUTHORIZED PERSONNEL

Name: _____ Manager, Safety Department: _____

Signature: _____ Phone: _____

is responsible for the overall program administration, including training of the workers. Administration of the program also shall include at least an annual review of the site Exposure Control Plan and retraining of employees as needed.

Supervisors

are responsible for ensuring that employees are familiar with and are following safety procedures outlined in the site Exposure Control Plan.

HAZARD RECOGNITION

It has been determined that the employees listed in Appendix B of this plan (site-specific) might be exposed to hazards of bloodborne pathogens while performing certain jobs or tasks in this facility. These employees are covered under the provisions of the OSHA bloodborne pathogens standard and this facility's Exposure Control Plan.

EXPOSURE CONTROL PROCEDURES

In all circumstances, Universal Precautions (see above) will be observed to prevent contact with blood and other potentially infectious materials, unless they interfere with the proper delivery of health care or would create a significant risk to the safety of the workers.

Engineering Controls

The OSHA bloodborne pathogens standard requires the use of engineering controls as a primary method for eliminating or controlling exposure to blood or other potentially infectious material. The following engineering controls will be used and enforced by all departmental supervisors:

1. Disposal of used needles, and other sharp wastes such as contaminated broken glass, into approved sharps containers.

2. Disposal of other regulated waste into approved infectious waste containers. (See Section E below [Waste Disposal] for procedures).

_____(FILL IN NAME)_____ is responsible for examining and maintaining all engineering controls on a regular basis. Records will be maintained for frequency of inspection and evaluation.

Required Work Practices (General)

1. Employees shall wash their hands immediately or as soon as possible after removal of gloves or other PPE, and after hand contact with blood or other potentially infectious materials.
2. All PPE must be removed immediately on leaving the work area or as soon as possible if overtly contaminated, and placed in an appropriately designated area or container for storage, washing, decontamination, or disposal.
3. Eating, drinking, smoking, applying cosmetics or lip balm, and handling contact lenses are prohibited in work areas where there is a potential for occupational exposure.
4. Food and drink shall not be stored in refrigerators, freezers, or cabinets where blood or other potentially infectious materials are stored or in areas of possible contamination.
5. All procedures involving blood or other potentially infectious materials will be done in a manner that minimizes splashing, spraying, and aerosolization of these substances.
6. If conditions are such that handwashing facilities are not available, antiseptic hand cleaners are to be used. Because this is an interim measure, employees are to wash hands at the first available opportunity.

Personal Protective Equipment

When there is potential for occupational exposure, employees will be provided and required to use PPE including — but not limited to — gloves, aprons, gowns, lab coats, head and foot coverings, and eye protectors (i.e., goggles, glasses with side shields, face shields). This equipment will be provided at no cost to employees. When necessary, hypoallergenic powderless or other alternative gloving will be provided to employees who are allergic to types normally provided.

Supplies may be obtained at the following locations:

_____

_____

Single use (disposable) gloves may not be decontaminated or washed for re-use.

Before leaving the work area, PPE (including laboratory coats) must be removed and disposed of properly, or placed into designated storage or laundry areas. Employees are not permitted to carry any type of PPE home for cleaning or other use.

PPE will be considered "appropriate" only if it does not permit blood or other potentially infectious materials to pass through or contact the employee's clothing, skin, mouth, or mucous membranes.

Listed below are types of PPE available for employee use, and circumstances under which it must be used:

Item	Procedure

Decontamination of PPE will be performed as follows:

Equipment	Cleaner/Disinfectant	Frequency

Housekeeping

1. Work surfaces shall be decontaminated with an appropriate disinfectant after completion of a procedure; when surfaces are overtly contaminated; immediately after any spill of blood or other potentially infectious materials; and at the end of the workshift.
2. Protective coverings such as plastic wrap, aluminum foil, or imperviously backed absorbent paper may be used to cover equipment and environmental surfaces. These coverings shall be removed and replaced as necessary (i.e., on contamination, at the end of the workday).
3. Equipment that might become contaminated with blood or other potentially infectious materials will be checked routinely and prior to servicing or shipping, and shall be decontaminated as necessary.
4. All bins, pails, cans, and similar receptacles intended for re-use that could become contaminated with blood or other potentially infectious materials shall be inspected, cleaned, and disinfected immediately or as soon as possible upon visible contamination. A regular cleaning schedule will be established and addressed elsewhere in this plan.
5. Broken glassware that might be contaminated shall not be picked up directly with the hands. It shall be cleaned using mechanical means such as a brush and dust pan, tongs, or forceps.
6. Reusable items contaminated with blood or other potentially infectious materials shall be decontaminated prior to washing and/or reprocessing.
7. It is the responsibility of _____ (FILL IN NAME) _____ to ensure that the work site is maintained in a clean and sanitary condition. Facilities will be cleaned and disinfected with an appropriate agent as required.

Waste Disposal

All infectious waste destined for disposal shall be placed in closeable, leakproof containers or bags that are color-coded or labeled as herein described. It shall be the responsibility of _____ (FILL IN NAME) _____ to ensure that waste is disposed of properly and that the following rules are observed.

1. If outside contamination of the container or bag is likely to occur, a second leakproof container or bag that is closeable and labeled or color-coded (as per OSHA specifications) will be placed over the outside of the first and closed to prevent leakage during handling, storage, and transport.
2. Reusable containers may not be opened, emptied, or cleaned manually or in any other manner that would pose the risk of percutaneous injury.
3. Disposal of contaminated PPE will be provided at no cost to employees.

Laundry

1. Laundry that has been contaminated with blood or other potentially infectious materials, or might contain contaminated sharps, will be handled as little as possible and with a minimum of agitation.
2. Contaminated laundry must be bagged at the location where it was used and shall not be sorted or rinsed in patient care areas.
3. Contaminated laundry shall be placed and transported in bags that are labeled or color-coded as herein described. Whenever this laundry is wet and presents the possibility for soaking or leaking through the bag, it will be placed and transported in leakproof bags.

4. Employees responsible for handling potentially contaminated laundry are required to wear protective gloves and other appropriate PPE to prevent occupational exposure during handling or sorting.
5. Laundering of PPE is to be provided by the employer at no cost to employees.
6. If laundry is shipped off site to a second facility that does not use Universal Precautions in its handling of all laundry, bags or containers with appropriate labeling and/or color-coding will be used to communicate the hazards associated with this material.
7. The person(s) responsible for ensuring the proper handling, storage, shipping, or cleaning of contaminated laundry is(are):

_____

_____

Communication of Hazards to Workers

1. Signs

   • Signs will be posted at the entrance to the following areas:

Work Area	Procedure

   • Signs will bear the legend described in the OSHA bloodborne pathogens standard (29 CFR 1910.1030).

2. Labels

   • Warning labels shall be affixed to containers of infectious waste; refrigerators and freezers containing blood and other potentially infectious materials; and other containers used to store or transport blood or other potentially infectious materials except as provided below.
   • Labels will bear the legend described in the OSHA bloodborne pathogens standard (29 CFR 1910.1030). They will be fluorescent orange or orange-red or predominantly so, with lettering or symbols in a contrasting color.
   • All labels will be an integral part of the container or will be affixed as close as safely possible to the container by string, wire, adhesive, or any other method that prevents their loss of unintentional removal.
   • Red bags or red containers may be substituted for labels on containers of infectious waste.
   • The person(s) responsible for ensuring that containers of biohazardous waste are properly labeled is(are):

_____

_____

3. Information and Training

   • All workers with occupational exposure will participate in exposure control training prior to their initial assignments and at least annually thereafter. This training will be free of charge to employees and scheduled during working hours.
   • The person(s) responsible for providing this training and coordinating the program is(are):

_____

_____

- At the end of each training session, employees will acknowledge their participation in the program by signing a form provided by the company, an example of which is found in Appendix C of this plan.

Employees will receive training in the following areas. A copy of the OSHA standard will be provided and its contents explained. Employees will be given:

- a general explanation of the epidemiology and symptoms of bloodborne diseases;
- an explanation of modes of transmission of bloodborne pathogens;
- an explanation of the site Exposure Control Plan and where to obtain a copy of it;
- an explanation of the appropriate methods for recognizing tasks and procedures that might involve exposure to blood or other potentially infectious materials;
- an explanation of the use and limitations of practices that will prevent or reduce exposure, including appropriate engineering controls, work practices, and PPE;
- information on PPE that addresses types available, proper use, location, removal, handling, decontamination, and/or disposal;
- an explanation of the basis for selection of PPE;
- information on the Hepatitis B vaccine, including information on its efficacy, safety, and the benefits of being vaccinated;
- information on the appropriate actions to take and persons to contact in event of an emergency;
- procedures to follow if an exposure incident occurs, including the method for reporting the incident;
- information on the medical follow-up that will be made available, and on medical counseling provided to exposed individuals;
- an explanation of signs, labels, and/or color coding; and
- a question-and-answer session with the trainer.

Medical Surveillance

1. Any employee who might be exposed to potentially infectious materials within this company will be offered, at no cost, a vaccination for Hepatitis B, unless the employee has had a previous vaccination or antibody testing reveals the employee to be immune. If an employee declines the vaccination, he or she must sign a waiver form. An example of this form is found in Appendix C of this plan.
2. Should an employee be exposed to a potentially infectious material (via needle stick, splash, etc.) post-exposure evaluations will be provided. A confidential medical evaluation and follow-up should include:
   - documentation of the route(s) of exposure, HBV and HIV antibody status of the source patient(s) (if known), and the circumstances under which the exposure occurred;
   - if the source patient can be determined and permission is obtained, collection and testing of the source patient's blood to determine the presence of HIV or HBV infection;
   - collection of blood from the exposed employee as soon as possible after the exposure incident for determination of HIV/HBV status. Actual antibody or antigen testing of the blood or serum sample may be done at that time or at a later date, if the employee so requests. Samples will be preserved for at least 90 days; and
   - follow-up of the exposed employee, including antibody or antigen testing, counseling, illness reporting, and safe and effective post-exposure prophylaxis, according to standard recommendations for medical practices.
3. The attending physician will be provided the following information:
   - a copy of the OSHA bloodborne pathogens standard and its appendices;
   - a description of the affected employee's duties as they relate to the employee's occupational exposure;
   - results of the source individual's blood testing, if available; and
   - all medical records, including vaccination records, relevant to the treatment of the employee.

4. The attending physician will provide a written opinion to this employer concerning the following:
   - the physician's recommended limitations on the employee's ability to receive the Hepatitis B vaccination;
   - a statement that the employee has been informed of the results of the medical evaluation and that the employee has been told about any medical conditions resulting from exposure to blood or other potentially infectious materials that require further evaluation or treatment; and
   - specific findings or diagnoses that are related to the employee's ability to receive the HBV vaccination. Any other findings and diagnoses shall remain confidential.
5. For each evaluation under this section, the company will obtain and provide the employee with a copy of the attending physician's written opinion within 15 days of the completion of the evaluation.

Record Keeping

1. Medical records will be kept for the length of the worker's employment plus 30 years. Records will be maintained at the following location(s):

   _____

   _____

2. Training records shall be kept for at least three (3) years. These records will be maintained at the following locations:

   _____

   _____

Appendix A

OSHA Standard for Bloodborne Pathogens
(29 CFR 1910.1030)

§1910.1030 Bloodborne pathogens

(a) Scope and Application. This section applies to all occupational exposure to blood or other potentially infectious materials as defined by paragraph (b) of this section.

(b) Definitions. For purposes of this section, the following shall apply:

"Assistant Secretary" means the Assistant Secretary of Labor for Occupational Safety and Health, or designated representative.

"Blood" means human blood, human blood components, and products made from human blood.

"Bloodborne Pathogens" means pathogenic microorganisms that are present in human blood and can cause disease in humans. These pathogens include, but are not limited to, hepatitis B virus (HBV) and human immunodeficiency virus (HIV).

"Clinical Laboratory" means a workplace where diagnostic or other screening procedures are performed on blood or other potentially infectious materials.

"Contaminated" means the presence or the reasonably anticipated presence of blood or other potentially infectious materials on an item or surface.

"Contaminated Laundry" means laundry which has been soiled with blood or other potentially infectious materials or may contain sharps.

"Contaminated Sharps" means any contaminated object that can penetrate the skin including, but not limited to, needles, scalpels, broken glass, broken capillary tubes, and exposed ends of dental wires.

"Decontamination" means the use of physical or chemical means to remove, inactivate, or destroy bloodborne pathogens on a surface or item to the point where they are no longer capable of transmitting infectious particles and the surface or item is rendered safe for handling, use, or disposal.

"Director" means the Director of the National Institute for Occupational Safety and Health, U.S. Department of Health and Human Services, or designated representative.

"Engineering Controls" means controls (e.g., sharps disposal containers, self-sheathing needles) that isolate or remove the bloodborne pathogens hazard from the workplace.

"Exposure Incident" means a specific eye, mouth, other mucous membrane, non-intact skin, or parenteral contact with blood or other potentially infectious materials that results from the performance of an employee's duties.

"Handwashing Facilities" means a facility providing an adequate supply of running potable water, soap and single use towels or hot air drying machines.

"Licensed Healthcare Professional" is a person whose legally permitted scope of practice allows him or her to independently perform the activities required by paragraph (f) Hepatitis B Vaccination and Post-exposure Evaluation and Follow-up.

"HBV" means hepatitis B virus.

"HIV" means human immunodeficiency virus.

"Occupational Exposure" means reasonably anticipated skin, eye, mucous membrane, or parenteral contact with blood or other potentially infectious materials that may result from the performance of an employee's duties.

"Other Potentially Infectious Materials" means (1) The following human body fluids: semen, vaginal secretions, cerebrospinal fluid, synovial fluid, pleural fluid, pericardial fluid, peritoneal fluid, amniotic fluid, saliva in dental procedures, any body fluid that is visibly contaminated with blood, and all body fluids in situations where it is difficult or impossible to differentiate between body fluids; (2) Any unfixed tissue or organ (other than intact skin) from a human (living or dead); and (3) HIV-containing cell or tissue cultures, organ cultures, and HIV- or HBV-containing culture medium or other solutions; and blood, organs, or other tissues from experimental animals infected with HIV or HBV.

"Parenteral" means piercing mucous membranes or the skin barrier through such events as needlesticks, human bites, cuts, and abrasions.

"Personal Protective Equipment" is specialized clothing or equipment worn by an employee for protection against a hazard. General work clothes (e.g., uniforms, pants, shirts or blouses) not intended to function as protection against a hazard are not considered to be personal protective equipment.

"Production Facility" means a facility engaged in industrial-scale, large-volume or high concentration production of HIV or HBV.

"Regulated Waste" means liquid or semi-liquid blood or other potentially infectious materials; contaminated items that would release blood or other potentially infectious materials in a liquid or semi-liquid state if compressed; items that are caked with dried blood or other potentially infectious materials and are capable of releasing these materials during handling; contaminated sharps; and pathological and microbiological wastes containing blood or other potentially infectious materials.

"Research Laboratory" means a laboratory producing or using research laboratory-scale amounts of HIV or HBV. Research laboratories may produce high concentrations of HIV or HBV but not in the volume found in production facilities.

"Source Individual" means any individual, living or dead, whose blood or other potentially infectious materials may be a source of occupational exposure to the employee. Examples include, but are not limited to, hospital and clinic patients; clients in institutions for the developmentally disabled; trauma victims; clients of drug and alcohol treatment facilities; residents of hospices and nursing homes; human remains; and individuals who donate or sell blood or blood components.

"Sterilize" means the use of a physical or chemical procedure to destroy all microbial life including highly resistant bacterial endospores.

"Universal Precautions" is an approach to infection control. According to the concept of Universal Precautions, all human blood and certain human body fluids are treated as if known to be infectious for HIV, HBV, and other bloodborne pathogens.

"Work Practice Controls" means controls that reduce the likelihood of exposure by altering the manner in which a task is performed (e.g., prohibiting recapping of needles by a two-handed technique).

(c) Exposure Control.

(1) "Exposure Control Plan." (i) Each employer having an employee(s) with occupational exposure as defined by paragraph (b) of this section shall establish a written Exposure Control Plan designed to eliminate or minimize employee exposure.

(ii) The Exposure Control Plan shall contain at least the following elements:

(A) The exposure determination required by paragraph (c)(2),

(B) The schedule and method of implementation for paragraphs (d) Methods of Compliance, (e) HIV and HBV Research Laboratories and Production Facilities, (f) Hepatitis B Vaccination and Post-Exposure Evaluation and Follow-up, (g) Com-

munication of Hazards to Employees, and (h) Recordkeeping, of this standard, and

(C) The procedure for the evaluation of circumstances surrounding exposure incidents as required by paragraph (f)(3)(i) of this standard.

(iii) Each employer shall ensure that a copy of the Exposure Control Plan is accessible to employees in accordance with 29 CFR 1910.20(e).

(iv) The Exposure Control Plan shall be reviewed and updated at least annually and whenever necessary to reflect new or modified tasks and procedures which affect occupational exposure and to reflect new or revised employee positions with occupational exposure.

(v) The Exposure Control Plan shall be made available to the Assistant Secretary and the Director upon request for examination and copying.

(2) "Exposure Determination." (i) Each employer who has an employee(s) with occupational exposure as defined by paragraph (b) of this section shall prepare an exposure determination. This exposure determination shall contain the following:

(A) A list of all job classifications in which all employees in those job classifications have occupational exposure;

(B) A list of job classifications in which some employees have occupational exposure, and

(C) A list of all tasks and procedures or groups of closely related task and procedures in which occupational exposure occurs and that are performed by employees in job classifications listed in accordance with the provisions of paragraph (c)(2)(i)(B) of this standard.

(ii) This exposure determination shall be made without regard to the use of personal protective equipment.

(d) Methods of Compliance.

(1) "General." Universal precautions shall be observed to prevent contact with blood or other potentially infectious materials. Under circumstances in which differentiation between body fluid types is difficult or impossible, all body fluids shall be considered potentially infectious materials.

(2) "Engineering and Work Practice Controls."

(i) Engineering and work practice controls shall be used to eliminate or minimize employee exposure. Where occupational exposure remains after institution of these controls, personal protective equipment shall also be used.

(ii) Engineering controls shall be examined and maintained or replaced on a regular schedule to ensure their effectiveness.

(iii) Employers shall provide handwashing facilities which are readily accessible to employees.

(iv) When provision of handwashing facilities is not feasible, the employer shall provide either an appropriate antiseptic hand cleanser in conjunction with clean cloth/paper towels or antiseptic towelettes. When antiseptic hand cleansers or towelettes are used, hands shall be washed with soap and running water as soon as feasible.

(v) Employers shall ensure that employees wash their hands immediately or as soon as feasible after removal of gloves or other personal protective equipment.

(vi) Employers shall ensure that employees wash hands and any other skin with soap and water, or flush mucous membranes with water immediately or as soon as feasible following contact of such body areas with blood or other potentially infectious materials.

(vii) Contaminated needles and other contaminated sharps shall not be bent, recapped, or removed except as noted in paragraphs (d)(2)(vii)(A) and (d)(2)(vii)(B) below. Shearing or breaking of contaminated needles is prohibited.

(A) Contaminated needles and other contaminated sharps shall not be bent, recapped or removed unless the employer can demonstrate that no alternative is feasible or that such action is required by a specific medical or dental procedure.

(B) Such bending, recapping or needle removal must be accomplished through the use of a mechanical device or one-handed technique.

(viii) Immediately or as soon as possible after use, contaminated reusable sharps shall be placed in appropriate containers until properly reprocessed. These containers shall be:

(A) puncture resistant;

(B) labeled or color-coded in accordance with this standard;

(C) leakproof on the sides and bottom; and

(D) in accordance with the requirements set forth in paragraph (d)(4)(ii)(E) for reusable sharps.

(ix) Eating, drinking, smoking, applying cosmetics or lip balm, and handling contact lenses are prohibited in work areas where there is a reasonable likelihood of occupational exposure.

(x) Food and drink shall not be kept in refrigerators, freezers, shelves, cabinets or on countertops or benchtops where blood or other potentially infectious materials are present.

(xi) All procedures involving blood or other potentially infectious materials shall be performed in such a manner as to minimize splashing, spraying, spattering, and generation of droplets of these substances.

(xii) Mouth pipetting/suctioning of blood or other potentially infectious materials is prohibited.

(xiii) Specimens of blood or other potentially infectious materials shall be placed in a container which prevents leakage during collection, handling, processing, storage, transport, or shipping.

(A) The container for storage, transport, or shipping shall be labeled or color-coded according to paragraph (g)(1)(i) and closed prior to being stored, transported, or shipped. When a facility utilizes Universal Precautions in the handling of all specimens, the labeling/color-coding of specimens is not necessary provided containers are recognizable as containing specimens. This exemption only applies while such specimens/containers remain within the facility. Labeling or color-coding in accordance with paragraph (g)(1)(i) is required when such specimens/containers leave the facility.

(B) If outside contamination of the primary container occurs, the primary container shall be placed within a second container which prevents leakage during handling, processing, storage, transport, or shipping and is labeled or color-coded according to the requirements of this standard.

(C) If the specimen could puncture the primary container, the primary container shall be placed within a secondary container which is puncture-resistant in addition to the above characteristics.

(xiv) Equipment which may become contaminated with blood or other potentially infectious materials shall be examined prior to servicing or shipping and shall be decontaminated as necessary, unless the employer can demonstrate that decontamination of such equipment or portions of such equipment is not feasible.

(A) A readily observable label in accordance with paragraph (g)(1)(i)(H) shall be attached to the equipment stating which portions remain contaminated.

(B) The employer shall ensure that this information is conveyed to all affected employees, the servicing representative, and/or the manufacturer, as appropriate, prior to handling, servicing, or shipping so that appropriate precautions will be taken.

(3) "Personal Protective Equipment."

(i) "Provision." When there is occupational exposure, the employer shall provide, at no cost to the employee, appropriate personal protective equipment such as, but not limited to, gloves, gowns, laboratory coats, face shields or masks and eye protection, and mouthpieces, resuscitation bags, pocket masks, or other ventilation devices. Personal protective equipment will be considered "appropriate" only if it does not permit blood or other potentially infectious materials to pass through to or reach the employee's work clothes, street clothes, undergarments, skin, eyes, mouth, or other mucous membranes under normal conditions of use and for the duration of time which the protective equipment will be used.

(ii) "Use." The employer shall ensure that the employee uses appropriate personal protective equipment unless the employer shows that the employee temporarily and briefly declined to use personal protective equipment when, under rare and extraordinary circumstances, it was the employee's professional judgment that in the specific instance its use would have prevented the delivery of health care or public safety services or would have posed an increased hazard to the safety of the worker or co-worker. When the employee makes this judgement, the circumstances shall be investigated and documented in order to determine whether changes can be instituted to prevent such occurrences in the future.

(iii) "Accessibility." The employer shall ensure that appropriate personal protective equipment in the appropriate sizes is readily accessible at the worksite or is issued to employees. Hypoallergenic gloves, glove liners, powderless gloves, or other similar alternatives shall be readily accessible to those employees who are allergic to the gloves normally provided.

(iv) "Cleaning, Laundering, and Disposal." The employer shall clean, launder, and dispose of personal protective equipment required by paragraphs (d) and (e) of this standard, at no cost to the employee.

(v) "Repair and Replacement." The employer shall repair or replace personal protective equipment as needed to maintain its effectiveness, at no cost to the employee.

(vi) If a garment(s) is penetrated by blood or other potentially infectious materials, the garment(s) shall be removed immediately or as soon as feasible.

(vii) All personal protective equipment shall be removed prior to leaving the work area.

(viii) When personal protective equipment is removed it shall be placed in an appropriately designated area or container for storage, washing, decontamination or disposal.

(ix) "Gloves." Gloves shall be worn when it can be reasonably anticipated that the employee may have hand contact with blood, other potentially infectious materials, mucous membranes, and non-intact skin; when performing vascular access procedures except as specified in paragraph (d)(3)(ix)(D); and when handling or touching contaminated items or surfaces.

(A) Disposable (single use) gloves such as surgical or examination gloves, shall be replaced as soon as practical when contaminated or as soon as feasible if they are torn, punctured, or when their ability to function as a barrier is compromised.

(B) Disposable (single use) gloves shall not be washed or decontaminated for re-use.

(C) Utility gloves may be decontaminated for reuse if the integrity of the glove is not compromised. However, they must be discarded if they are cracked, peeling, torn, punctured, or exhibit other signs of deterioration or when their ability to function as a barrier is compromised.

(D) If an employer in a volunteer blood donation center judges that routine gloving for all phlebotomies is not necessary then the employer shall:

(1) Periodically reevaluate this policy;

(2) Make gloves available to all employees who wish to use them for phlebotomy;

(3) Not discourage the use of gloves for phlebotomy; and

(4) Require that gloves be used for phlebotomy in the following circumstances:

(i) When the employee has cuts, scratches, or other breaks in his or her skin;

(ii) When the employee judges that hand contamination with blood may occur, for example, when performing phlebotomy on an uncooperative source individual; and

(iii) When the employee is receiving training in phlebotomy.

(x) "Masks, Eye Protection, and Face Shields." Masks in combination with eye protection devices, such as goggles or glasses with solid side shields, or chin-length face shields, shall be worn whenever splashes, spray, spatter, or droplets of blood or other potentially infectious materials may be generated and eye, nose, or mouth contamination can be reasonably anticipated.

(xi) "Gowns, Aprons, and Other Protective Body Clothing." Appropriate protective clothing such as, but not limited to, gowns, aprons, lab coats, clinic jackets, or similar outer garments shall be worn in occupational exposure situations. The type and characteristics will depend upon the task nd degree of exposure anticipated.

(xii) Surgical caps or hoods and/or shoe covers or boots shall be worn in instances when gross contamination can reasonably be anticipated (e.g., autopsies, orthopaedic surgery).

(4) "Housekeeping."

(i) "General." Employers shall ensure that the worksite is maintained in a clean and sanitary condition. The employer shall determine and implement an appropriate written schedule for cleaning and method of decontamination based upon the location within the facility, type of surface to be cleaned, type of soil present, and tasks or procedures being performed in the area.

(ii) All equipment and environmental and working surfaces shall be cleaned and decontaminated after contact with blood or other potentially infectious materials.

(A) Contaminated work surfaces shall be decontaminated with an appropriate disinfectant after completion of procedures; immediately or as soon as feasible when surfaces are overtly contaminated or after any spill of blood or other potentially infectious materials; and at the end of the work shift if the surface may have become contaminated since the last cleaning.

(B) Protective coverings, such as plastic wrap, aluminum foil, or imperviously-backed absorbent paper used to cover equipment and environmental surfaces, shall be removed and replaced as soon as feasible when they become overtly contaminated or at the end of the workshift if they may have become contaminated during the shift.

(C) All bins, pails, cans, and similar receptacles intended for reuse which have a reasonable likelihood for becoming contaminated with blood or other potentially infectious materials shall be inspected and decontaminated on a regularly scheduled basis and cleaned and decontaminated immediately or as soon as feasible upon visible contamination.

(D) Broken glassware which may be contaminated shall not be picked up directly with the hands. It shall be cleaned up using mechanical means, such as a brush and dust pan, tongs, or forceps.

(E) Reusable sharps that are contaminated with blood or other potentially infectious materials shall not be stored or processed in a manner that requires employees to reach by hand into the containers where these sharps have been placed.

(iii) Regulated Waste.

(A) Contaminated Sharps Discarding and Containment.

(1) Contaminated sharps shall be discarded immediately or as soon as feasible in containers that are:

(A) Closable;

(B) Puncture resistant;

(C) Leakproof on sides and bottom; and

(D) Labeled or color-coded in accordance with paragraph (g)(1)(i) of this standard.

(2) During use, containers for contaminated sharps shall be:

(A) Easily accessible to personnel and located as close as is feasible to the immediate area where sharps are used or can be reasonably anticipated to be found (e.g., laundries);

(B) Maintained upright throughout use; and

(C) Replaced routinely and not be allowed to overfill.

(3) When moving containers of contaminated sharps from the area of use, the containers shall be:

(A) Closed immediately prior to removal or replacement to prevent spillage or protrusion of contents during handling, storage, transport, or shipping;

(B) Placed in a secondary container if leakage is possible. The second container shall be:

(i) Closable;

(ii) Constructed to contain all contents and prevent leakage during handling, storage, transport, or shipping; and

(iii) Labeled or color-coded according to paragraph (g)(1)(i) of this standard.

(4) Reusable containers shall not be opened, emptied, or cleaned manually or in any other manner which would expose employees to the risk of percutaneous injury.

(B) Other Regulated Waste Containment.

(1) Regulated waste shall be placed in containers which are:

(A) Closable;

(B) Constructed to contain all contents and prevent leakage of fluids during handling, storage, transport, or shipping;

(C) labeled or color-coded in accordance with paragraph (g)(1)(i) of this standard; and

(D) Closed prior to removal to prevent spillage or protrusion of contents during handling, storage, transport, or shipping.

(2) If outside contamination of the regulated waste container occurs, it shall be placed in a second container. The second container shall be:

(A) Closable;

(B) Constructed to contain all contents and prevent leakage of fluids during handling, storage, transport or shipping;

(C) Labeled or color-coded in accordance with paragraph (g)(1)(i) of this standard; and

(D) Closed prior to removal to prevent spillage or protrusion of contents during handling, storage, transport, or shipping.

(E) Disposal of all regulated waste shall be in accordance with applicable regulations of the United States, States and Territories, and political subdivisions of States and Territories.

(iv) "Laundry."

(A) Contaminated laundry shall be handled as little as possible with a minimum of agitation.

(1) Contaminated laundry shall be bagged or con-

tainerized at the location where it was used and shall not be sorted or rinsed in the location of use.

(2) Contaminated laundry shall be placed and transported in bags or containers labeled or color-coded in accordance with paragraph (g)(1)(i) of this standard. When a facility utilizes Universal Precautions in the handling of all soiled laundry, alternative labeling or color-coding is sufficient if it permits all employees to recognize the containers as requiring compliance with Universal Precautions.

(3) Whenever contaminated laundry is wet and presents a reasonable likelihood of soak-through of or leakage from the bag or container, the laundry shall be placed and transported in bags or containers which prevent soak-through and/or leakage of fluids to the exterior.

(B) The employer shall ensure that employees who have contact with contaminated laundry wear protective gloves and other appropriate personal protective equipment.

(C) When a facility ships contaminated laundry off-site to a second facility which does not utilize Universal Precautions in the handling of all laundry, the facility generating the contaminated laundry must place such laundry in bags or containers which are labeled or color-coded in accordance with paragraph (g)(1)(i).

(e) HIV and HBV Research Laboratories and Production Facilities.

(1) This paragraph applies to research laboratories and production facilities engaged in the culture, production, concentration, experimentation, and manipulation of HIV and HBV. It does not apply to clinical or diagnostic laboratories engaged solely in the analysis of blood, tissues, or organs. These requirements apply in addition to the other requirements of the standard.

(2) Research laboratories and production facilities shall meet the following criteria:

(i) "Standard Microbiological Practices." All regulated waste shall either be incinerated or decontaminated by a method such as autoclaving known to effectively destroy bloodborne pathogens.

(ii) "Special Practices."

(A) Laboratory doors shall be kept closed when work involving HIV or HBV is in progress.

(B) Contaminated materials that are to be decontaminated at a site away from the work area shall be placed in a durable, leakproof, labeled or color-coded container that is closed before being removed from the work area.

(C) Access to the work area shall be limited to authorized persons. Written policies and procedures shall be established whereby only persons who have been advised of the potential biohazard, who meet any specific entry requirements, and who comply with all entry and exit procedures shall be allowed to enter the work areas and animal rooms.

(D) When other potentially infectious materials or infected animals are present in the work area or containment module, a hazard warning sign incorporating the universal biohazard symbol shall be posted on all access doors. The hazard warning sign shall comply with paragraph (g)(1)(ii) of this standard.

(E) All activities involving other potentially infectious materials shall be conducted in biological safety cabinets or other physical-containment devices within the containment module. No work with these other potentially infectious materials shall be conducted on the open bench.

(F) Laboratory coats, gowns, smocks, uniforms, or other appropriate protective clothing shall be used in the work area and animal rooms. Protective clothing shall not be worn outside of the work area and shall be decontaminated before being laundered.

(G) Special care shall be taken to avoid skin contact with other potentially infectious materials. Gloves shall be worn when handling infected animals and when making hand contact with other potentially infectious materials is unavoidable.

(H) Before disposal all waste from work areas and from animal rooms shall either be incinerated or decontaminated by a method such as autoclaving known to effectively destroy bloodborne pathogens.

(I) Vacuum lines shall be protected with liquid disinfectant traps and high-efficiency particulate air (HEPA) filters or filters of equivalent or superior efficiency and which are checked routinely and maintained or replaced as necessary.

(J) Hypodermic needles and syringes shall be used only for parenteral injection and aspiration of fluids from laboratory animals and diaphragm bottles. Only needle-locking syringes or disposable syringe-needle units (i.e., the needle is integral to the syringe) shall be used for the injection or aspiration of other potentially infectious materials. Extreme caution shall be used when handling needles and syringes. A needle shall not be bent, sheared, replaced in the sheath or guard, or removed from the syringe following use. The needle and syringe shall be promptly placed in a puncture-resistant container and autoclaved or decontaminated before reuse or disposal.

(K) All spills shall be immediately contained and cleaned up by appropriate professional staff or others properly trained and equipped to work with potentially concentrated infectious materials.

(L) A spill or accident that results in an exposure incident shall be immediately reported to the laboratory director or other responsible person.

(M) A biosafety manual shall be prepared or adopted and periodically reviewed and updated at least annually or more often if necessary. Personnel shall be advised of potential hazards, shall be required to read instructions on practices and procedures, and shall be required to follow them.

(iii) "Containment Equipment."

(A) Certified biological safety cabinets (Class I, II, or III) or other appropriate combinations of personal protection or physical containment devices, such as special protective clothing, respirators, centrifuge safety cups, sealed centrifuge rotors, and containment caging for animals, shall be used for all activities with other potentially infectious materials that pose a threat of exposure to droplets, splashes, spills, or aerosols.

(B) Biological safety cabinets shall be certified when installed, whenever they are moved and at least annually.

(3) "HIV and HBV research laboratories shall meet the following criteria:"

(i) Each laboratory shall contain a facility for hand washing and an eye wash facility which is readily available within the work area.

(ii) An autoclave for decontamination of regulated waste shall be available.

(4) "HIV and HBV production facilities shall meet the following criteria:"

(i) The work areas shall be separated from areas that are open to unrestricted traffic flow within the building. Passage through two sets of doors shall be the basic requirement for entry into the work area from access corridors or other contiguous areas. Physical separation of the high-containment work area from access corridors or other areas or activities may also be provided by a double-doored clothes-change room (showers may be included), airlock, or other access facility that requires passing through two sets of doors before entering the work area.

(ii) The surfaces of doors, walls, floors and ceilings in the work area shall be water resistant so that they can be easily cleaned. Penetrations in these surfaces shall be sealed or capable of being sealed to facilitate decontamination.

(iii) Each work area shall contain a sink for washing hands and a readily available eye wash facility. The sink shall be foot, elbow, or automatically operated and shall be located near the exit door of the work area.

(iv) Access doors to the work area or containment module shall be self-closing.

(v) An autoclave for decontamination of regulated waste shall be available within or as near as possible to the work area.

(vi) A ducted exhaust-air ventilation system shall be provided. This system shall create directional airflow that draws air into the work area through the entry area. The exhaust air shall not be recirculated to any other area of the building, shall be discharged to the outside, and shall be dispersed away from occupied areas and air intakes. The proper direction of the airflow shall be verified (i.e., into the work area).

(5) "Training Requirements." Additional training requirements for employees in HIV and HBV research laboratories and HIV and HBV production facilities are specified in paragraph (g)(2)(ix).

(f) *Hepatitis B Vaccination and Post-exposure Evaluation and Follow-up.*

(1) "General." (i) The employer shall make available the hepatitis B vaccine and vaccination series to all employees who have occupational exposure, and post-exposure evaluation and follow-up to all employees who have had an exposure incident.

(ii) The employer shall ensure that all medical evaluations and procedures including the hepatitis B vaccine and vaccination series and post-exposure evaluation and follow-up, including prophylaxis, are:

(A) Made available at no cost to the employee;

(B) Made available to the employee at a reasonable time and place;

(C) Performed by or under the supervision of a licensed physician or by or under the supervision of another licensed healthcare professional; and

(D) Provided according to recommendations of the U.S. Public Health Service current at the time these evaluations and procedures take place, except as specified by this paragraph (f).

(iii) The employer shall ensure that all laboratory tests are conducted by an accredited laboratory at no cost to the employee.

(2) "Hepatitis B Vaccination." (i) Hepatitis B vaccination shall be made available after the employee has received the training required in paragraph (g)(2)(vii)(I) and within 10 working days of initial assignment to all employees who have occupational exposure unless the employee has previously received the complete hepatitis B vaccination series, antibody testing has revealed that the employee is immune, or the vaccine is contraindicated for medical reasons.

(ii) The employer shall not make participation in a prescreening program a prerequisite for receiving hepatitis B vaccination.

(iii) If the employee initially declines hepatitis B vaccination but at a later date while still covered under the standard decides to accept the vaccination, the employer shall make available hepatitis B vaccination at that time.

(iv) The employer shall assure that employees who decline to accept hepatitis B vaccination offered by the employer sign the statement in Appendix A.

(v) If a routine booster dose(s) of hepatitis B vaccine is recommended by the U.S. Public Health Service at a future date, such booster dose(s) shall be made available in accordance with section (f)(1)(ii).

(3) "Post-exposure Evaluation and Follow-up." Following a report of an exposure incident, the employer shall make immediately available to the exposed employee a confidential medical evaluation and follow-up, including at least the following elements:

(i) Documentation of the route(s) of exposure, and the circumstances under which the exposure incident occurred;

(ii) Identification and documentation of the source individual, unless the employer can establish that identification is infeasible or prohibited by state or local law;

(A) The source individual's blood shall be tested as soon as feasible and after consent is obtained in order to determine HBV and HIV infectivity. If consent is not obtained, the employer shall establish that legally required consent cannot be obtained. When the source individual's consent is not required by law, the source individual's blood, if available, shall be tested and the results documented.

(B) When the source individual is already known to be infected with HBV or HIV, testing for the source individual's known HBV or HIV status need not be repeated.

(C) Results of the source individual's testing shall be made available to the exposed employee, and the employee shall be informed of applicable laws and regulations concerning disclosure of the identity and infectious status of the source individual.

(iii) Collection and testing of blood for HBV and HIV serological status;

(A) The exposed employee's blood shall be collected as soon as feasible and tested after consent is obtained.

(B) If the employee consents to baseline blood collection, but does not give consent at that time for HIV serologic testing, the sample shall be preserved for at least 90 days. If, within 90 days of the exposure incident, the employee elects to have the baseline sample tested, such testing shall be done as soon as feasible.

(iv) Post-exposure prophylaxis, when medically indicated, as recommended by the U.S. Public Health Service;

(v) Counseling; and

(vi) Evaluation of reported illnesses.

(4) "Information provided to the healthcare professional." (i) The employer shall ensure that the healthcare professional responsible for the employee's Hepatitis B vaccination is provided a copy of this regulation.

(ii) The employer shall ensure that the healthcare professional evaluating an employee after an exposure incident is provided the following information:

(A) A copy of this regulation;

(B) A description of the exposed employee's duties as they relate to the exposure incident;

(C) Documentation of the route(s) of exposure and circumstances under which exposure occurred;

(D) Results of the source individual's blood test, if available; and

(E) All medical records relevant to the appropriate treatment of the employee including vaccination status which are the employer's responsibility to maintain.

(5) "Healthcare professional's written opinion." The employer shall obtain and provide the employee with a copy of the evaluating healthcare professional's written opinion within 15 days of the completion of the evaluation.

(i) The healthcare professional's written opinion for Hepatitis B vaccination shall be limited to whether Hepatitis B vaccination is indicated for an employee, and if the employee has received such vaccination.

(ii) The healthcare professional's written opinion for post-exposure evaluation and follow-up shall be limited to the following information:

(A) That the employee has been informed of the results of the evaluation; and

(B) That the employee has been told about any medical conditions resulting from exposure to blood or other potentially infectious materials which require further evaluation or treatment.

(iii) All other findings or diagnoses shall remain confidential and shall not be included in the written report.

(6) "Medical Recordkeeping." Medical records required by this standard shall be maintained in accordance with paragraph (h)(1) of this section.

(g) Communication of Hazards to Employees.

(1) "Labels and Signs." (i) Labels.

(A) Warning labels shall be affixed to containers of regulated waste, refrigerators and freezers containing blood or other potentially infectious material; and other containers used to store, transport or ship blood or other potentially infectious materials, except as provided in paragraph (g)(1)(i)(E), (F) and (G).

(B) Labels required by this section shall include the following legend:

[For the universal biohazard symbol, please refer to Chapter 5 (Figure 2) of the AIHA Biosafety Manual, 2nd Edition. Include the name of the infectious agent; special requirements for entering the area; and the name and telephone number of the laboratory director or other responsible person.]

(C) These labels shall be fluorescent orange or orange-red or predominantly so, with lettering and symbols in a contrasting color.

(D) Labels shall be affixed as close as feasible to the container by string, wire, adhesive, or other method that prevents their loss or unintentional removal.

(E) Red bags or red containers may be substituted for labels.

(F) Containers of blood, blood components, or blood products that are labeled as to their contents and have been released for transfusion or other clinical use are exempted from the labeling requirements of paragraph (g).

(G) Individual containers of blood or other potentially infectious materials that are placed in a labeled container during storage, transport, shipment or disposal are exempted from the labeling requirement.

(H) Labels required for contaminated equipment shall be in accordance with this paragraph and shall also state which portions of the equipment remain contaminated.

(I) Regulated waste that has been decontaminated need not be labeled or color-coded.

(ii) Signs.

(A) The employer shall post signs at the entrance to work areas specified in paragraph (e), HIV and HBV Research Laboratory and Production Facilities, which shall bear the following legend:

[For the universal biohazard symbol, please refer to Chapter 5 (Figure 2) of the AIHA Biosafety Manual, 2nd Edition. Include the name of the infectious agent; special requirements for entering the area; and the name and telephone number of the laboratory director or other responsible person.]

(B) These signs shall be fluorescent orange-red or predominantly so, with lettering and symbols in a contrasting color.

(2) "Information and Training." (i) Employers shall ensure that all employees with occupational exposure participate in a training program which must be provided at no cost to the employee and during working hours.

(ii) Training shall be provided as follows:

(A) At the time of initial assignment to tasks where occupational exposure may take place;

(B) Within 90 days after the effective date of the standard; and

(C) At least annually thereafter.

(iii) For employees who have received training on bloodborne pathogens in the year preceding the effective date of the standard, only training with respect to the provisions of the standard which were not included need be provided.

(iv) Annual training for all employees shall be provided within one year of their previous training.

(v) Employers shall provide additional training when changes such as modification of tasks or procedures affect the employee's occupational exposure. The additional training may be limited to addressing the new exposures created.

(vi) Material appropriate in content and vocabulary to educational level, literacy, and language of employees shall be used.

(vii) The training program shall contain at a minimum the following elements:

(A) An accessible copy of the regulatory text of this standard and an explanation of its contents;

(B) A general explanation of the epidemiology and symptoms of bloodborne diseases;

(C) An explanation of the modes of transmission of bloodborne pathogens;

(D) An explanation of the employer's exposure control plan and the means by which the employee can obtain a copy of the written plan;

(E) An explanation of the appropriate methods for recognizing tasks and other activities that may involve exposure to blood and other potentially infectious materials;

(F) An explanation of the use and limitations of methods that will prevent or reduce exposure including appropriate engineering controls, work practices, and personal protective equipment;

(G) Information on the types, proper use, location, removal, handling, decontamination and disposal of personal protective equipment;

(H) An explanation of the basis for selection of personal protective equipment;

(I) Information on the hepatitis B vaccine, including information on its efficacy, safety, method of administration, the benefits of being vaccinated, and that the vaccine and vaccination will be offered free of charge;

(J) Information on the appropriate actions to take and persons to contact in an emergency involving blood or other potentially infectious materials;

(K) An explanation of the procedure to follow if an exposure incident occurs, including the method of reporting the incident and the medical follow-up that will be made available;

(L) Information on the post-exposure evaluation and follow-up that the employer is required to provide for the employee following an exposure incident;

(M) An explanation of the signs and labels and/or color coding required by paragraph (g)(1); and

(N) An opportunity for interactive questions and answers with the person conducting the training session.

(viii) The person conducting the training shall be knowledgeable in the subject matter covered by the elements contained in the training program as it relates to the workplace that the training will address.

(ix) Additional Initial Training for Employees in HIV and HBV Laboratories and Production Facilities. Employees in HIV or HBV research laboratories and HIV or HBV production facilities shall receive the following initial training in addition to the above training requirements.

(A) The employer shall assure that employees demonstrate proficiency in standard microbiological practices and techniques and in the practices and operations specific to the facility before being allowed to work with HIV or HBV.

(B) The employer shall assure that employees have prior experience in the handling of human pathogens or tissue cultures before working with HIV or HBV.

(C) The employer shall provide a training program to employees who have no prior experience in handling human pathogens. Initial work activities shall not include the handling of infectious agents. A progression of work activities shall be assigned as techniques are learned and proficiency is developed. The employer shall assure that employees participate in work activities involving infectious agents only after proficiency has been demonstrated.

(h) Recordkeeping.

(1) "Medical Records." (i) The employer shall establish and maintain an accurate record for each employee with occupational exposure, in accordance with 29 CFR 1910.20.

(ii) This record shall include:

(A) The name and social security number of the employee;

(B) A copy of the employee's hepatitis B vaccination status including the dates of all the hepatitis B vaccinations and any medical records relative to the employee's ability to receive vaccination as required by paragraph (f)(2);

(C) A copy of all results of examinations, medical testing, and follow-up procedures as required by paragraph (f)(3);

(D) The employer's copy of the healthcare professional's written opinion as required by paragraph (f)(5); and

(E) A copy of the information provided to the healthcare professional as required by paragraphs (f)(4)(ii)(B), (C) and (D).

(iii) Confidentiality. The employer shall ensure that employee medical records required by paragraph (h)(1) are:

(A) Kept confidential; and

(B) Not disclosed or reported without the employee's express written consent to any person within or outside the workplace except as required by this section or as may be required by law.

(iv) The employer shall maintain the records required by paragraph (h) for at least the duration of employment plus 30 years in accordance with 29 CFR 1910.20.

(2) "Training Records." (i) Training records shall include the following information:

(A) The dates of the training sessions;

(B) The contents or a summary of the training sessions;

(C) The names and qualifications of persons conducting the training; and

(D) The names and job titles of all persons attending the training sessions.

(ii) Training records shall be maintained for 3 years from the date on which the training occurred.

(3) "Availability." (i) The employer shall ensure that all records required to be maintained by this section shall be made available upon request to the Assistant Secretary and the Director for examination and copying.

(ii) Employee training records required by this paragraph shall be provided upon request for examination and copying to employees, to employee representatives, to the Director, and to the Assistant Secretary.

(iii) Employee medical records required by this paragraph shall be provided upon request for examination and copying to the subject employee, to anyone having written consent of the subject employee, to the Director, and to the Assistant Secretary in accordance with 29 CFR 1910.20.

(4) "Transfer of Records." (i) The employer shall comply with the requirements involving transfer of records set forth in 29 CFR 1910.20(h).

(ii) If the employer ceases to do business and there is no successor employer to receive and retain the records for the prescribed period, the employer shall notify the Director, at least three months prior to their disposal and transmit them to the Director, if required by the Director to do so, within that three month period.

(i) Dates.

(1) "Effective Date." The standard shall become effective on March 6, 1992.

(2) The Exposure Control Plan required by paragraph (c) of this section shall be completed on or before May 5, 1992.

(3) Paragraph (g)(2) Information and Training and (h) Recordkeeping shall take effect on or before June 4, 1992.

(4) Paragraphs (d)(2) Engineering and Work Practice Controls, (d)(3) Personal Protective Equipment, (d)(4) Housekeeping, (e) HIV and HBV Research Laboratories and Production Facilities, (f) Hepatitis B Vaccination and Post-Exposure Evaluation and Follow-up, and (g)(1) Labels and Signs, shall take effect July 6, 1992.

[56 FR 64004, Dec. 06, 1991, as amended at 57 FR 12717, April 13, 1992; 57 FR 29206, July 1, 1992]

(Appendices for this standard are not included in this version.)

Appendix B

Occupationally Exposed Workers (Site-Specific)

Name	Position	Duties

Appendix C

Employee Forms

This appendix includes forms for bloodborne pathogens training and employee hepatitis B declination.

Bloodborne Pathogens Training

On _____(DATE)_____, I attended company-provided training on bloodborne pathogens. Covered in this training were:

a. The OSHA bloodborne pathogens standard (copy provided) and an explanation of its contents;
b. A general explanation of the epidemiology and symptoms of bloodborne diseases;
c. An explanation of modes of transmission of bloodborne pathogens;
d. An explanation of the site Exposure Control Plan;
e. An explanation of the appropriate methods of recognizing tasks and procedures that might involve exposure to blood or other potentially infectious materials;
f. An explanation of the use and limitations of practices that will prevent or reduce exposure, including engineering controls, work practices, and personal protective equipment;
g. Information on types, proper use, location, removal, handling, decontamination, and/or disposal of personal protective equipment;
h. The basis for selecting personal protective equipment;
i. Information on the hepatitis B vaccine, its efficacy, safety, and the benefits of being vaccinated;
j. Information on the how to respond to emergencies;
k. Procedures to follow if an exposure incident occurs, including the method of reporting the incident;
l. The medical follow-up that will be made available. Also, information on medical counseling provided to exposed individuals;
m. An explanation of signs, labels, and/or color-coding; and
n. A question-and-answer session with the trainer.

_____   _____

(Supervisor/Trainer Initials)   (Employee's Signature)

175

Employee Hepatitis B Declination

STATEMENT:

I understand that, due to my occupational exposure to blood or other potentially infectious materials, I might be at risk of acquiring hepatitis B virus (HBV) infection. I have been given the opportunity to be vaccinated with hepatitis B vaccine, at no charge to myself; however, I decline hepatitis B vaccination at this time. I understand that by declining this vaccine, I continue to be at risk of acquiring hepatitis B, a serious disease. If in the future I continue to have occupational exposure to blood or other potentially infectious materials and I want to be vaccinated with hepatitis B vaccine, I can receive the vaccination series at no charge to me.

_____

(Signature)

_____

(Date)

AIHA PUBLICATIONS

(Prices are listed as member/nonmember and are subject to change.)

Basic Industrial Hygiene Principles

Basic Industrial Hygiene: A Training Manual .... $18/$28
Engineering Field Reference Manual .... $20/$30
Inorganic Lead Guidance Document .... $345/$395
Noise & Hearing Conservation Manual .... $41/$51
Quality Assurance Manual for Industrial
   Hygiene Chemistry .... $35/$45
   (Chapter 11 only) .... $7/$10

Computers/Communication

The American Industrial Hygiene Association:
   Its History and Personalities 1939-1990 .... $30/$35
The AIHA Journal 10-Year Index (1984-1993) .... $20/$25
Computers in Health and Safety .... $35/$40
Exploring the Dangerous Trades: The Auto-
   biography of Alice Hamilton, M.D. .... $20/$25
Industrial Hygiene Auditing:
   A Manual for Practice .... $38/$48
Responding to Community Outrage: Strategies
   for Effective Risk Communication .... $20/$25
Risk = Hazard + Outrage: A Formula for
   Effective Risk Communication
   (Two-Tape Training Video) .... $275/$395*
What in the World is an Industrial Hygienist?
   (Tape) .... $25/$40

Environmental Quality

ANSI/AIHA Z9.3 Standard for Spray Finishing
   Operations .... $25/$30
ANSI/AIHA Z9.5 Standard for Laboratory
   Ventilation .... $28/$35
The Industrial Hygienist's Guide to Indoor
   Air Quality Investigations .... $16/$24
The Practitioner's Approach to Indoor Air Quality
   Investigations: Proceedings of the Indoor Air
   Quality International Symposium .... $36/$44
IAQ and HVAC Workbook, Second Edition .... $42/$45
Industrial Ventilation Workbook, Third Edition ..... $42/$45
Laboratory Ventilation Workbook, 2nd Edition ..... $42/$45

Ergonomics

Ergonomics Guide Series:
   • An Ergonomics Guide to VDT Workstations ... $12/$16
   • Dynamic Measures of Low Back
     Performance .... $10/$12
   • Cumulative Trauma Disorders of the Hand
     and Wrist, An Ergonomics Guide .... $10/$12
   • An Ergonomics Guide to Hand Tools .... $12/$16
Manual Material Handling: Understanding
   and Preventing Back Trauma .... $32/$42

Exposure Assessment

Emergency Response Planning Guideline
   Series .... $14/$20 per set

LOGAN Workplace Exposure Evaluation
   System .... $150/$225
Nonionizing Radiation Guide Series:
   • Extremely Low Frequency Electric and
     Magnetic Fields .... $24/$32
   • General Concepts .... $10/$14
   • Radio-Frequency and Microwave Radiation,
     Second Edition .... $18/$25
   • Ultraviolet Radiation .... $12/$18
Occupational Exposure, Toxic Properties, and
   Work Practice Guidelines for Fiber Glass .... $18/$25
Odor Thresholds for Chemicals with Established
   Occupational Health Standards .... $38/$48
A Strategy for Occupational Exposure
   Assessment .... $40/$50
Workplace Environmental Exposure Level
   Guide Series .... $12/$18 per set

OSHA Compliance

Confined Space Entry:
   An AIHA Protocol Guide .... $12/$18
Hazard Communication:
   An AIHA Protocol Guide .... $12/$18

Protective Clothing/Equipment

Chemical Protective Clothing, Volume 1 .... $45/$60
Chemical Protective Clothing, Volume 2:
   Product and Performance Information .... $60/$75
Respiratory Protection: A Manual and
   Guideline, Second Edition .... $40/$50

Risk Identification/Control

Arc Welding and Your Health: Information for
   Welding .... $10/$15
Biosafety Reference Manual,
   Second Edition .... $35/$45
Welding Health and Safety Resource
   Manual .... $15/$22

Sampling/Instrumentation

Direct-Reading Colorimetric Indicator
   Tubes Manual, Second Edition .... $24/$32
Manual of Recommended Practice for
   Combustible Gas Indicators and Portable
   Direct-Reading Hydrocarbon Detectors,
   Second Edition .... $24/$32
Manual of Recommended Practice for
   Portable Direct-Reading Carbon Monoxide
   Indicators .... $15/$25
Particle Sampling Using Cascade Impactors:
   Some Practical Application Issues .... $12/$16
Sampling for Environmental Lead .... $7/$10

***For information about other Peter Sandman
videos, call (703) 849-8888.**